Heart Failure with Reduced Ejection Fraction

Editor

ASAD GHAFOOR

CARDIOLOGY CLINICS

www.cardiology.theclinics.com

November 2023 • Volume 41 • Number 4

ELSEVIER

1600 John F. Kennedy Boulevard • Suite 1800 • Philadelphia, Pennsylvania, 19103-2899

http://www.theclinics.com

CARDIOLOGY CLINICS Volume 41, Number 4
November 2023 ISSN 0733-8651, ISBN-13: 978-0-443-18195-5

Editor: Joanna Gascoine
Developmental Editor: Isha Singh

Cardiology Clinics (ISSN 0733-8651) is published quarterly by Elsevier Inc., 360 Park Avenue South, New York, NY 10010-1710. Months of issue are February, May, August, and November. Business and Editorial Offices: 1600 John F. Kennedy Blvd., Ste. 1800, Philadelphia, PA 19103-2899. Customer Service Office: 3251 Riverport Lane, Maryland Heights, MO 63043. Periodicals postage paid at New York, NY and additional mailing offices. Subscription prices are $377.00 per year for US individuals, $743.00 per year for US institutions, $100.00 per year for US students and residents, $468.00 per year for Canadian individuals, $932.00 per year for Canadian institutions, $490.00 per year for international individuals, $932.00 per year for international institutions, $100.00 per year for Canadian students/residents and $220.00 per year for international students/residents. To receive student/resident rate, orders must be accompanied by name of affiliated institution, data of term, and the *signature* of program/residency coordinator on institution letterhead. Orders will be billed at individual rate until proof of status is received. Foreign air speed delivery is included in all *Clinics* subscription prices. All prices are subject to change without notice. **POSTMASTER:** Send address changes to *Cardiology Clinics*, Elsevier Health Sciences Division, Subscription Customer Service, 3251 Riverport Lane, Maryland Heights, MO 63043. **Customer Service: 1-800-654-2452 (U.S. and Canada); 314-447-8871 (outside U.S. and Canada). Fax: 314-447-8029. E-mail: journalscustomerservice-usa@elsevier.com (for print support); journalsonlinesupport-usa@elsevier.com (for online support).**

Reprints. For copies of 100 or more, of articles in this publication, please contact the Commercial Reprints Department, Elsevier Inc., 360 Park Avenue South, New York, NY 10010-1710. Tel.: 212-633-3874; Fax: 212-633-3820; E-mail: reprints@elsevier.com.

Cardiology Clinics is also published in Spanish by McGraw-Hill Interamericana Editores S. A., P.O. Box 5-237, 06500, Mexico D. F., Mexico; in Portuguese by Reichmann and Alfonso Editores Rio de Janeiro, Brazil; and in Greek by Dimitrios P. Lagos, 8 Pondon Street, GR115-28 Ilissia, Greece.

Cardiology Clinics is covered in *MEDLINE/PubMed (Index Medicus), Excerpta Medica, The Cumulative Index to Nursing and Allied Health Literature* (CINAHL).

Contributors

EDITORIAL BOARD

JAMIL A. ABOULHOSN, MD, FACC, FSCAI
Director, Ahmanson/UCLA Adult Congenital Heart Center, Streisand/American Heart Association Endowed Chair, Divisions of Cardiology and Pediatric Cardiology, David Geffen School of Medicine at UCLA, Los Angeles, California, USA

DAVID M. SHAVELLE, MD, FACC, FSCAI
Director, Department of Cardiology Director, Interventional Cardiology MemorialCare Heart and Vascular Institute (MHVI), Long Beach Medical Center, Long Beach, California, USA

AUDREY H. WU, MD, MPH
Associate Professor, Advanced Heart Failure and Transplant Program, Division of Cardiovascular Medicine, Department of Medicine, University of Michigan, Ann Arbor, Michigan, USA

EDITOR

ASAD GHAFOOR, MD, MS
Program Director, Advanced Heart Failure and Transplant Fellowship, Aurora St. Luke's Medical Center, Milwaukee, Wisconsin, USA

AUTHORS

KEITH AARONSON MD
Department of Internal Medicine, Division of Cardiovascular Medicine, University of Michigan, Cardiovascular Center, Ann Arbor, Michigan, USA

JOSE AGUILAR, MD
Division of Cardiovascular Medicine, The Mount Sinai Health System, New York, New York, USA

LARRY A. ALLEN, MD, MHS
Division of Cardiology, Department of Medicine, University of Colorado School of Medicine, Aurora, Colorado, USA

MATTHEW B. AMDAHL, MD, PhD
Fellow, Department of Cardiovascular Diseases, Mayo Clinic, Rochester, Minnesota, USA

MICHAEL H. BEASLEY, MD
Assistant Professor of Medicine (Heart Failure and Transplant Cardiology), Section of Cardiovascular Medicine, Yale New Haven Hospital, New Haven, Connecticut, USA

ABBAS BITAR, MD
Department of Internal Medicine, Division of Cardiovascular Medicine, University of Michigan, Cardiovascular Center, Ann Arbor, Michigan, USA

KHADIJAH BREATHETT, MD, MS
Division of Cardiovascular Medicine, Indiana University, Indianapolis, Indiana, USA

JAVED BUTLER, MD, MPH, MBA
Department of Medicine, University of Mississippi Medical Center, Jackson, Mississippi, USA; Baylor Scott & White Research Institute, Dallas, Texas, USA

JOHANNA CONTRERAS, MD
Division of Cardiovascular Medicine, The
Mount Sinai Health System, New York, New
York, USA

JERRY D. ESTEP, MD
Robert and Suzanne Tomsich Department of
Cardiology, Section of Heart Failure and
Cardiac Transplant Medicine, Cleveland Clinic,
Weston, Florida, USA

ALEJANDRO FOLCH, MD
Division of Cardiovascular Medicine, The
Mount Sinai Health System, New York, New
York, USA

KENDALL FREE, BS
Department of Biofunction Research, Tokyo
Medical and Dental University, Tokyo, Japan

STEPHEN J. GREENE, MD
Division of Cardiology, Department of
Medicine, Duke University Hospital, Durham,
North Carolina, USA

KASHVI GUPTA, MD, MPH
Saint Luke's Mid America Heart Institute,
University of Missouri-Kansas City, Kansas
City, Missouri, USA

JIUN-RUEY HU, MD, MPH
Section of Cardiovascular Medicine, Yale
School of Medicine, New Haven, Connecticut,
USA

ONYEDIKA ILONZE, MD, MS
Division of Cardiovascular Medicine, Indiana
University, Indianapolis, Indiana, USA

**ARSHAD JAHANGIR, MD, FACC, FAHA,
FHRS**
Aurora Cardiovascular and Thoracic Services,
Center for Advanced Atrial Fibrillation
Therapies, Aurora Sinai/Aurora St. Luke's
Medical Centers, Advocate Aurora Health,
Milwaukee, Wisconsin, USA

MOHSIN KHAN, MD
Aurora Cardiovascular and Thoracic Services,
Center for Advanced Atrial Fibrillation
Therapies, Aurora Sinai/Aurora St. Luke's
Medical Centers, Advocate Aurora Health,
Milwaukee, Wisconsin, USA

MUHAMMAD SHAHZEB KHAN, MD, MSc
Division of Cardiology, Department of
Medicine, Duke University Hospital, Durham,
North Carolina, USA

EMILY FRYMAN LOWE, MD
Department of Medicine, University of
Colorado School of Medicine, Aurora,
Colorado, USA

IOANNIS MASTORIS, MD
Cardiology Division, Department of Medicine,
Massachusetts General Hospital, Boston,
Massachusetts, USA

DAN D. MATLOCK, MD, MPH
Adult and Child Center for Outcomes Research
and Delivery Science (ACCORDS), University
of Colorado School of Medicine, Children's
Hospital Colorado, Aurora, Colorado, USA

SULA MAZIMBA, MD, MPH
Division of Cardiovascular Medicine, University
of Virginia, Charlottesville, Virginia, USA

ABDULELAH NUQALI, MBBS
Section of Cardiovascular Medicine, Yale New
Haven Hospital, New Haven, Connecticut, USA

MICHAEL J. PIENTA, MD, MS
Department of Cardiac Surgery, Michigan
Medicine, University of Michigan, Ann Arbor,
Michigan, USA

ROOPA RAO, MD
Division of Cardiovascular Medicine, Indiana
University, Indianapolis, Indiana, USA

YOGESH N.V. REDDY, MBBS
Assistant Professor, Department of
Cardiovascular Diseases, Mayo Clinic,
Rochester, Minnesota, USA; University
Hospitals Medical Center, Cleveland, Ohio,
USA

RALPH J. RIELLO, PharmD
Clinical and Translational Research
Accelerator, Yale School of Medicine, New
Haven, Connecticut, USA

MATTHEW A. ROMANO, MD
Department of Cardiac Surgery, Michigan
Medicine, University of Michigan, Ann Arbor,
Michigan, USA

ANDREW J. SAUER, MD
Saint Luke's Mid America Heart Institute,
University of Missouri-Kansas City, Kansas
City, Missouri, USA

ALEXANDRA N. SCHWANN, MD
Department of Internal Medicine, Yale New
Haven Hospital, New Haven, Connecticut, USA

DAVID SNIPELISKY, MD
Robert and Suzanne Tomsich Department of
Cardiology, Section of Heart Failure and
Cardiac Transplant Medicine, Cleveland Clinic,
Weston, Florida, USA

VARUN SUNDARAM, MBBS
Associate Professor, Louis Stokes Cleveland
VA Medical Center, Case Western Reserve
University, Cleveland, Ohio, USA

KHAWAJA M. TALHA, MBBS
Department of Medicine, University of
Mississippi Medical Center, Jackson,
Mississippi, USA

JIA WEI TAN, MD
Division of Nephrology, Stanford University
School of Medicine, Palo Alto, California, USA

ELIZABETH O. TINUOYE, MSc
Division of Cardiovascular Medicine, The
Mount Sinai Health System, New York, New
York, USA

Contents

> Minoritized racial and ethnic groups have the highest incidence, prevalence, and hospitalization rate for heart failure. Despite improvement in medical therapies and overall survival, the morbidity and mortality of these groups remain elevated. The reasons for this disparity are multifactorial, including social determinant of health (SDOH) such as access to care, bias, and structural racism. These same factors contributed to higher rates of COVID-19 infection among minoritized racial and ethnic groups. In this review, we aim to explore the lessons learned from the COVID-19 pandemic and its interconnection between heart failure and SDOH. The pandemic presents a window of opportunity for achieving greater equity in the health care of all vulnerable populations.

> Treatment of heart failure with reduced ejection fraction (HFrEF) has benefitted from a proliferation of new medications and devices. These treatments carry important clinical benefits, but also come with costs relevant to payers, providers, and patients. Patient out-of-pocket costs have been implicated in the avoidance of medical care, nonadherence to medications, and the exacerbation of health care disparities. In the absence of major health care policy and payment redesign, high-quality HFrEF care delivery requires transparent integration of cost considerations into system design, patient-clinician interactions, and medical decision making.

> The conventional sequence of guideline-directed medical therapy (GDMT) initiation in heart failure with reduced ejection fraction (HFrEF) assumes that the effectiveness and tolerability of GDMT agents mirror their order of discovery, which is not true. In this review, the authors discuss flexible GDMT sequencing that should be permitted in special populations, such as patients with bradycardia, chronic kidney disease, or atrial fibrillation. Moreover, the initiation of certain GDMT medications may enable tolerance of other GDMT medications. Most importantly, the achievement of partial doses of all four pillars of GDMT is better than achievement of target dosing of only a couple.

Frailty affects half of all patients with heart failure with reduced ejection fraction (HFrEF) and carries a ~2-fold increased risk of mortality. The relationship between frailty and HFrEF is bidirectional, with one condition exacerbating the other. Paradoxical to their higher clinical risk, frail patients with HFrEF are more often undertreated due to concerns over medication-related adverse clinical events. However, current evidence suggests consistent safety of HF medical therapies among older frail patients with HFrEF. A multidisciplinary effort is necessary for the appropriate management of these high-risk patients which focuses on the optimization of known beneficial therapies with a goal-directed effort toward improving quality of life.

Obesity has been long recognized as a risk factor for the development of heart failure, but recent evidence suggests obesity is more typically associated with heart failure with preserved ejection fraction as opposed to heart failure with reduced ejection fraction (HFrEF). Nevertheless, numerous studies have found that obesity modulates the presentation and progression of HFrEF and may contribute to the development of HFrEF in some patients. Although obesity has definite negative effects in HFrEF patients, the effects of intentional weight loss in HFrEF patients with obesity have been poorly studied.

Life-threatening dysrhythmias remain a significant cause of mortality in patients with nonischemic cardiomyopathy (NICM). Implantable cardioverter-defibrillators (ICD) effectively reduce mortality in patients who have survived a life-threatening arrhythmic event. The evidence for survival benefit of primary prevention ICD for patients with high-risk NICM on guideline-directed medical therapy is not as robust, with efficacy questioned by recent studies. In this review, we summarize the data on the risk of life-threatening arrhythmias in NICM, the recommendations, and the evidence supporting the efficacy of primary prevention ICD, and highlight tools that may improve the identification of patients who could benefit from primary prevention ICD implantation.

Successful remote patient monitoring depends on bidirectional interaction between patients and multidisciplinary clinical teams. Invasive pulmonary artery pressure monitoring has been shown to reduce heart failure (HF) hospitalizations, facilitate guideline-directed medical therapy optimization, and improve quality of life. Cardiac implantable electronic device-based multiparameter monitoring has shown encouraging results in predicting future HF-related events. Potential expanded indications for remote monitoring include guideline-directed medical therapy optimization, application to specific populations, and subclinical detection of HF. Voice analysis, inferior vena cava diameter monitoring, and artificial intelligence–based remote electrocardiogram show potential to gain some merit in remote patient monitoring in HF.

Transcatheter mitral valve repair should be considered for patients with severe secondary mitral regurgitation with symptomatic heart failure with reduced ejection fraction for symptom improvement and survival benefit. Patients with a higher severity of secondary mitral regurgitation relative to the degree of left ventricular dilation are more likely to benefit from transcatheter mitral valve repair. A multidisciplinary Heart Team should participate in patient selection for transcatheter mitral valve therapy.

Cardiogenic shock is a multisystem pathology that carries a high mortality rate, and initial pharmacotherapies include the use of vasopressors and inotropes. These agents can increase myocardial oxygen consumption and decrease tissue perfusion that can oftentimes result in a state of refractory cardiogenic shock for which temporary mechanical circulatory support can be considered. Numerous support devices are available, each with its own hemodynamic blueprint. Defining a patient's hemodynamic profile and understanding the phenotype of cardiogenic shock is important in device selection. Careful patient selection incorporating a multidisciplinary team approach should be utilized.

Heart failure (HF) is a progressive disease. It is estimated that more than 250,000 patients suffer from advanced HF with reduced ejection fraction refractory to medical therapy. With limited donor pool for heart transplant, continue flow left ventricle assist device (LVAD) is a lifesaving treatment option for patients with advanced HF. This review will provide an update on indications, contraindications, and associated adverse events for LVAD support with a summary of the current outcomes data.

CARDIOLOGY CLINICS

SERIES OF RELATED INTEREST

Heart Failure Clinics
Available at: https://www.heartfailure.theclinics.com/
Cardiac Electrophysiology Clinics
Available at: https://www.cardiacep.theclinics.com/
Interventional Cardiology Clinics
Available at: https://www.interventional.theclinics.com/

Preface
Turning Heart Failure into Heart Success

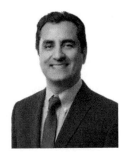

Asad Ghafoor, MD, MS, FACC
Editor

Cardiovascular disease has remained a leading cause of demise for both sexes. Clinicians have been able to delay the onset of disease and help people live longer. However, longevity has come with an increasing population of heart failure (HF) patients. Luckily, an expanding set of tools has allowed us to manage these patients through different stages of HF. But our challenges extend beyond methods of treatment, and a humanistic approach is required to address the whole problem, not just the pathophysiology of the disease. We hope the collection of articles in this issue of *Cardiology Clinics* will sum up some of the challenges and future aspirations in the clinical community.

In a postpandemic world, we have learned and relearned many lessons. Poignant among these is the disparity witnessed in health care delivery to minoritized groups. Dr Breathhett and colleagues eloquently discuss the influence of social determinants of health. These include access to care, bias, and structured racism. The authors point out fewer referrals to cardiac rehab programs, ventricular assist devices, transplants, and percutaneous valve therapies for African American, Hispanic, and Asian patients. This work is ongoing, and we hope will be reflected in policymaking in the future. The pandemic presents an opportunity for prioritizing access to care, particularly for those with the highest morbidity and mortality risk.

We cannot ignore the economic aftermath of HF. Dr Allen and colleagues discuss the need for transparency and real-time cost data integration to allow for fluent clinical decision making. While new medical therapies exist and hold much promise, they are yet to become affordable for most patients. As reported by the authors, costs of lost economic productivity account for one-fifth of the American economy. Moreover, medical debt is the leading cause of bankruptcy in the United States. As clinicians, we need to advocate for the financial security of our patients. Health care cannot and should not be a costly privilege.

Speaking of newer therapies, how has the paradigm shifted? Dr Beasley and colleagues delineate specific phenotypes where the patient's clinical presentation dictates the sequencing of medical treatments. In an era of personalized medicine, this is precisely the approach that our patients expect. In a figure that speaks a thousand words, the authors have summarized well the new paradigm of guideline-directed medical therapy (GDMT).

Aging with HF poses challenges like frailty. Dr Khan and colleagues describe the consequences of a clinician's perception of their patient's frailty. Such patients are less likely to be placed on appropriate GDMT, less likely to be referred to cardiac rehabilitation programs, and less likely to be offered life-prolonging advanced therapies and remote monitoring systems to avoid recurrent hospitalizations. Frail patients are more likely to be women. To complicate this matter, objective determinants of frailty have long been lacking, but there appears to be momentum behind the increasing use of the Clinical Frailty Scale in HF clinical trials.

Another unfortunate pairing with HF is obesity. Dr Reddy and colleagues discuss the statistical paradox whereby obesity is associated with better outcomes in heart failure with reduced ejection fraction (HFrEF). We lack data regarding the influence of intentional weight loss in patients with reduced ejection fraction. There is nothing to indicate that it is harmful. Furthermore, there is increasing enthusiasm surrounding GLP-1 agonists for weight loss. However, two randomized clinical trials of Liraglutide in reduced ejection fraction patients did not show improved clinical outcomes. Therefore, while use in diabetes and atherosclerotic cardiovascular disease patients is supported, data do not support benefit in HFrEF patients, reinforcing the need for dedicated trials with GLP-1 agonists in patients with HF.

Dr Jahangir revisits an old debate by examining the utility of implantable defibrillators in nonischemic cardiomyopathy. Contemporary medical and device therapies likely drive the diminishing mortality benefit. As the authors report, this observation is more prominent in older age groups. The Seattle Proportional Risk Model (SPRM) is a valuable tool for clinical decision making. In a study referenced by the authors, the simultaneous use of the Seattle Heart Failure Model enhanced SPRM's predictive ability. When both scores were above the median, there was a statistically significant reduction in all-cause mortality with ICD implantation.

In the advanced spectrum of HF patients, there is a significant necessity for reducing HF hospitalizations. In the GUIDE-HF trial, the only FDA-approved implantable hemodynamic pulmonary artery pressure sensor did not show a reduction in all-cause mortality and HF events. However, a pre–COVID-19 analysis indicated a possible benefit. Dr Sauer and colleagues discuss the vast array of tools available for remote monitoring and the data behind them. A key element of remote patient monitoring is its ability to reflect changes postintervention. Illustrated examples include favorable hemodynamic changes post–left ventricular assist device, post–gastric bypass surgery, and after initiation of a new medical therapy like SGLT2i. One can only postulate that the possibilities are endless. Imagine the integration of information between devices. The so-called Internet of Things could bring a new technological revolution to HF.

In recent years, FDA approval for percutaneous mitral intervention has played a role in clamping the influence of secondary mitral regurgitation in HF hospitalizations. Analysis of the COAPT trial showed that patients with disproportionately severe mitral regurgitation benefited the most, with a number needed to treat (NNT) to prevent death from any cause of 5.9 patients at 24 months. To put this in perspective, Entresto had an NNT of 40 patients at 27 months in the PARADIGM-HF trial. Dr Pienta and colleagues summarize the progress so far and reflect that further work is needed to clarify which patients with advanced HF would benefit from transcatheter mitral valve therapies.

Acute decompensated HF and cardiogenic shock remain the Achilles heel of HFrEF. Management requires a thorough know-how of percutaneous mechanical support options, which has been an ever-changing landscape, not just because of increasing levels of support available but also because of the increasing use of the axillary artery approach. Dr Estep and colleagues describe how defining the hemodynamic profile is vital in device selection. Managing cardiogenic shock has become an art, where anticipating the timing of escalating support is often the pivotal ingredient to saving lives. More recently, in the Detroit Cardiogenic Shock Initiative, cardiogenic shock teams have been shown to improve survival. What is frequently needed is a prompt goal-directed multidisciplinary effort. With enough practice, one envisions a shock team running like a well-oiled machine. For a minority of patients, the solution is more durable support, which is well illustrated by Dr Aaronson and colleagues in the article "When all else fails, try this: The HeartMate III Left Ventricular Assist Device."

Ultimately, all these contributions by our authors are an effort to integrate the different aspects of HF care. In clinical practice, the best care for our patients dictates compassion, empathy, and lengthy discussions about tailoring available therapies to their wishes and beliefs. From a clinical decision-making standpoint, it is crucial to remind oneself that there comes a point in these discussions where we are past the concept of right and wrong, and what becomes more paramount is what is acceptable to our patients. In the words of Rumi, "Somewhere beyond right and wrong, there is a garden. I will meet you there."

Asad Ghafoor, MD, MS
Program Director
Advance Heart Failure & Transplant Fellowship
Aurora St. Luke's Medical Center
Milwaukee, WI 53215

E-mail address:
asad.ghafoor@aah.org

Heart Failure with Reduced Ejection Fraction and COVID-19, when the Sick Get Sicker

Unmasking Racial and Ethnic Inequities During a Pandemic

Johanna Contreras, MD[a], Elizabeth O. Tinuoye, MSc[a], Alejandro Folch, MD[a],
Jose Aguilar, MD[a], Kendall Free, BS[b], Onyedika Ilonze, MD, MS[c],
Sula Mazimba, MD, MPH[d], Roopa Rao, MD[c], Khadijah Breathett, MD, MS[c],*

KEYWORDS

• COVID-19 • Heart failure • Racial disparities • Ethnic disparities

KEY POINTS

- The COVID-19 pandemic illustrated the important relationship between social determinants of health and heart failure outcomes among minoritized racial and ethnic communities.
- Health care accessibility is a major challenge for minoritized racial and ethnic groups. These challenges are further exacerbated by policies that fail to address social determinants of health.
- Supporting studies that engage community-based participatory research and implementation science may lead to equity in heart failure care among minoritized racial and ethnic groups.

INTRODUCTION

Health care disparities are greatest for minoritized racial and ethnic groups and have worsened with the COVID-19 pandemic.[1] In 2020, Black patients were overrepresented in COVID-19 death statistics, with twice the expected total of deaths based on population size.[2] Black and Hispanic populations had a reduced life expectancy in 2021 and 2022 compared to White patients, related to COVID-19.[3] Moreover, American Indian populations experienced a decrease in life expectancy due to the COVID-19 pandemic.[4]

Similarly, risks of developing heart failure (HF) are greater in some minoritized racial and ethnic groups. Disparities in the treatment and recognition of precursors of HF may contribute to differences in HF presentation by race and ethnicity.[5] Hypertension is one of the main etiologies of HF and remains worse treated to control among Black and Mexican patients compared to White patients.[6] Black individuals have the highest prevalence of HF at 3.6%[7] and more than twice the risk of developing HF before the age of 65 compared to White women and men.[8] Latino/a/x and White men and women have a similar prevalence of HF.[7] However, abnormal left ventricular structure and function have been observed at younger ages in Latino/a/x individuals than White individuals.[7,9,10] Due to underreporting, there is limited information on the

[a] Division of Cardiovascular Medicine, The Mount Sinai Health System, 1190 5th Avenue, 1st Floor, New York, NY 10029, USA; [b] Department of Biofunction Research, Tokyo Medical and Dental University, 1-5-45 Yushima, Bunkyo-ku, Tokyo 113-8510, Japan; [c] Division of Cardiovascular Medicine, Indiana University, 1800 North Capitol Avenue, Indianapolis, IN 46202, USA; [d] Division of Cardiovascular Medicine, University of Virginia, 1215 Lee Street, Charlottesville, VA 22908-0158, USA

* Corresponding author.

E-mail address: kbreath@iu.edu

Cardiol Clin 41 (2023) 491–499
https://doi.org/10.1016/j.ccl.2023.06.006

prevalence of HF in the American Indian population.[7,11,12] In addition, minoritized racial and ethnic groups are less likely to be prescribed guideline-directed medical therapy (GDMT) and nonpharmacological therapies.[5,13]

COVID-19 influenced outcomes for patients with HF. Hospitalizations for HF with reduced ejection fraction (HFrEF) are often associated with increased mortality.[14] However, attempts to reduce hospitalizations do not necessarily equate reduced mortality. Multiple studies of the U.S. health care policy have demonstrated that attempting to reduce needed hospitalizations results in higher mortality.[15] Similarly, during the initial years of the COVID-19 pandemic, HF hospitalizations decreased inappropriately.[16] Data suggests that patients delayed and forwent hospital care out of concern for increased risk of COVID-19 in waiting rooms and in over-populated areas.[17] The full ramifications of delayed care and treatment are still forthcoming. In this review, we describe the interplay between HF, COVID-19, and outcomes for minoritized racial and ethnic groups, and propose strategies to improve access for these patients.

COVID-19 Unmasking Health Care Disparities

COVID-19 disproportionately affected minoritized racial and ethnic communities and lower resourced communities.[3,18,19] COVID-19 was declared a global public health emergency on March 11, 2020, by the World Health Organization (WHO),[20] and had catastrophic consequences since that time. Between March 1, 2020 and January 2, 2021 the excess death rate was higher among non-Hispanic Black populations (208.4 deaths per 100,000) than non-Hispanic White or Hispanic/Latinx populations (157.0 and 139.8 deaths per 100,000, respectively).[3] The COVID-19 pandemic unmasked significant differences in health care delivery.[21]

COVID-19 highlighted how intricately race, ethnicity, gender, and socioeconomic position impact the overall health of individuals and the community.[22,23] Vaccine hesitancy was simplistically mislabeled as a blanket reason for low initial receipt of COVID-19 vaccine among minoritized racial and ethnic populations and populations with lower socioeconomic resources. National work led by Dr. Boyd and others helped identify how systemic racism contributed to the low receipt of COVID-19.[24] Major issues included an untrustworthy medical system and unequitable access to care.[18,19] Patients were unsure of the effectiveness of vaccines in their population groups. Misinformation was prevalent. Patients were disadvantaged for lack of broadband internet, lack of knowledge of how to sign-up on electronic schedules that were frequently full, lack of primary care health professional relationships, lack of readily available transportation, lack of flexible jobs allowing sick d/d to visit health care professionals, and lack of funds to support childcare and or/travel for appointments.[25] A disproportionate amount of these burdens were upon minoritized racial and ethnic groups and women.

The pandemic furthered conversations relating to social determinants of health (SDOH). SDOH include education access and quality, health care and quality, neighborhood and built environment, social and community context, and economic stability.[26] SDOH are now recognized as being responsible for 50% or more of health care outcomes, higher than attribution for health behaviors.[27] The confluence of SDOH with COVID-19 resulted in communities being overburdened with disease and worse outcomes.[28] During the pandemic the social ills of society took center stage in the media. Many became aware of the importance of addressing SDOH to improve health outcomes beyond COVID-19, such as HF.

SDOH greatly impacted HF outcomes among minoritized racial and ethnic groups.[5] Education is associated with health literacy among patients with HF[29]; health literacy is associated with worse outcomes among patients with HF.[30] Due to redlining and structural racism, minoritized racial and ethnic groups have systematically worse access to good schools, financial and social support systems to obtain college education.[31–33] For years, health care access and quality have been robustly detailed as inequitable for minoritized racial and ethnic groups compared to White populations.[34,35] Despite deriving similar benefits from guideline directed therapy, African American patients are less likely than White patients to receive cardiac resynchronization therapy (CRT).[36,37] African American, Hispanic and Asian patients receive fewer physician referrals for cardiac exercise training and lower participation in cardiac rehabilitation than White patients.[38–40] A similar trend can also be seen in other therapies such as VAD, transplants and percutaneous mitral valve repair (TMVr).[5] Access to insurance has helped improve some disparities among patients with HF such as heart transplants,[41] but many remain in respect to access to other devices and therapies.[42–45] Related to redlining, neighborhood deprivation is associated with 12% increase in incident HF, [46] and food deserts are associated with increased HF risk, which are more prevalent among minoritized racial and ethnic communities.

SDOH must be addressed to reduce racial and ethnic HF disparities.[47]

Pathophysiology Between Heart Failure and COVID-19

Although the social context may be the most important for understanding racial and ethnic disparities in HF in relation to COVID-19, it is also important to contextualize how COVID-19 contributes to HF across racial and ethnic groups. COVID-19 can cause direct and indirect cardiomyocyte damage leading to HF. COVID-19 infection causes endothelial cell activation and dysfunction in macro and microcirculation resulting in thrombi formation and organ injury. Endotheliopathy causes vasoconstriction and vascular injury triggering thrombus formation from platelet hyperreactivity.[48] About 25% to 50% autopsy specimens have demonstrated the presence of the virus in subendothelium and pericytes.[49] Hypoxemia from respiratory infection, along with increased oxygen demand causes stress and weakening of cardiomyocytes.

The acute phase of severe COVID infection is associated with the release of pro-inflammatory cytokines such as interleukins, tumor necrosis factors, interferons. This attracts inflammatory cells and the dysregulated immune system causes cytotoxicity and organ damage.[50] Cardiac biomarkers such as troponin are usually elevated and portends worse prognosis. Cardiomyocytes have increased expression of angiotensin-converting enzyme 2 receptors. The virus attaches to these receptors to gain entry to the tissue. Imaging studies have shown myocardial inflammation even in asymptomatic patients.[51] Myocarditis from COVID-19 could be from direct invasion or from the heightened immune response. In addition, stress cardiomyopathy has been increasingly seen with COVID-19 infection with the reported incidence of about 7% during the early part of the pandemic.[52] Right HF alone can be seen in patients with severe pulmonary involvement or in patients with acute large pulmonary embolism. Diastolic HF physiology can be a sequel of COVID infection or could be from the progression of subclinical dysfunction from inflammation, fibrosis, and myocardial cell injury.

Relationship Between Heart Failure and COVID-19 Outcomes

HF in itself is also associated with poor outcomes with COVID-19 infection including an increase in mortality, intensive care utilization, and severity of infection. In a large database analysis of greater than 90,000 patients with diagnosis of COVID-19, history of HF was associated with increased mortality. In chronic stable HF, patients 30-day and 90-day mortality was 8.0% and 9.0% respectively, and patients with worsening HF had highest mortality of 15.6% and 16.5%.[53] Another study reported 1 in 3 in patients with HFrEF died and attributed this high rate of mortality to comorbid conditions and sociodemographic position.[54] Patients recovered from COVID-19 hospitalization with no prior history of HF are also at increased risk of developing de novo HF. In the national cohort COVID collaborative study, authors noted a 45% higher hazard of incident HF.[55] Although the exact etiology of this association is not clear, shared pathophysiology is thought to be the cause.

COVID-19 was associated with the reduction in HF hospitalizations. A retrospective study of an urban hospital in northern Philadelphia revealed a 10% decrease after the start of the COVID pandemic, in a period comprising January 2019 to November 2020.[56] Similar findings were observed in a large medical center in Mississippi, where HF hospitalizations declined by 50% after the first diagnosed case in the state, with a further decline after that date.[16] Furthermore, a nationwide study in United Kingdom saw a 46% decline in HF hospitalization post-pandemic when compared to pre-pandemic data, and this was accompanied by increased community mortality.[57]

Multiple theories have been proposed to explain the decline in HF hospitalizations. This decrease in hospitalizations has been attributed to a decreased rate of presentation to the hospital secondary to patient's fears of contracting COVID-19 while receiving medical care during the pandemic.[16] In addition, the volume of COVID-19 cases overwhelmed the health care system and is thought to have led to decreased ability to deal with non-COVID related conditions, including certain cardiovascular conditions such as HF.[58]

Increased cardiovascular mortality associated with COVID-19 was notably more common among minoritized racial and ethnic groups.[59] A U.S. National Center for Health Statistics study revealed that Black, Hispanic, and Asian populations each experienced an approximate 20% increase in heart disease deaths, compared to 2% for non-Hispanic White populations from March to August 2020, compared to the same months in 2019.[59] While the COVID-19 pandemic was associated with an increased cardiovascular disease mortality in all ethnic groups, another retrospective nationwide study in the US revealed that Black individuals had 3-fold higher rates of excess CVD mortality (13.8%) compared to White individuals (5.1%).[60] Excess mortality due to HF was also higher in Black individuals, with a 9.1% increase in 2020 compared to a 0% increase in White individuals.

Relationship Between Heart Failure Disparities and Access to Care

Inadequate access to care remains a key contributor to higher rates of death with COVID-19 and HF for minoritized racial and ethnic groups. Pre-existing problems in U.S. health care delivery were worsened during the pandemic when access to health care professionals was limited to emergencies.[61] Factors such as clinical inertia, cost of care, lack of insurance or underinsurance, clinician bias and structural racism disproportionately limit access to care for minoritized patients and can worsen during a pandemic.[13,35] Low prescribing patterns of HF GDMT exist overall but under the prescription of HF GDMT therapy is worse in Black patients who have a higher HF disease burden than other populations.[13,62,63] For multiple centers, telemedicine did not facilitate major changes in GDMT prescribing patterns during the pandemic and in some cases resulted in lower prescribing of GDMT.[64,65] While this is variable across centers, it is important to recognized that telemedicine may not benefit under resourced communities substantially if barriers to broadband internet are not also addressed,[66] which disproportionately impacts minoritized racial and ethnic groups.

Inadequate insurance is an established barrier to HF care and an SDOH. U.S. health care policies which expanded access to health care insurance such as the Affordable Care Act (ACA) Medicaid Expansion have been associated with increased prescribing of one form of HF GDMT in Hispanic patients,[42] increased listing for heart transplant among Black patients, [41] but has not increased delivery rates across minoritized racial and ethnic groups to proportionate levels of disease prevalence. Furthermore, this policy was not associated with improvement in the delivery of cardiac resynchronization therapies,[44] nor ventricular assist devices (VAD)[43] across racial and ethnic groups. This does not negate the importance of adequate insurance but stresses the need for insurance that is broadly accepted, appropriately reimbursed, and not associated with additional biased care.

Clinician bias and structural racism are associated with reduced access to HF care for minoritized racial and ethnic groups. In both national and single-center studies, Black patients have been less likely than White patients to receive care by a cardiologist when admitted for HF.[67,68]

Black patients have consistently been less likely to receive advanced HF therapies than White patients in national databanks and multi-center studies.[69,70] A national study of heart failure health care professionals randomized to two patient vignettes differing only by race demonstrated that Black race was associated with lower likelihood of allocating a patient to heart transplant due to concerns of trust and adherence despite similar presentation as a White patient; social history and adherence were the most significant factors contributing to not allocating heart transplant.[71] Bias against minoritized groups can disadvantage them during the allocation of life-saving HF therapies. During public health emergencies when health care professionals have heightened stress and less time to process, this is the perfect setting for biased care to occur since there is reliance on automatic or habitual decision-making.[72] Minoritized racial and ethnic groups may be at higher risk of receiving biased care. This may explain the worse delivery of GDMT for minoritized racial and ethnic patients with acute myocardial infarction during the COVID-19 pandemic compared to White patients[73] as summarized in **Fig. 1**.

Additional studies are needed to test strategies to correct major etiologies of inequitable HF care delivery such as clinical inertia, social determinants of health (eg, underinsurance), bias, and structural racism. This will lead to better delivery of HF care and better preparedness during future public health emergencies.

STEPS TO ADDRESS BARRIERS
Clinical Inertia May Be Addressed Through Systematic Changes in the Care Delivery Process

Recently, data from the Safety, tolerability, and efficacy of up-titration of guideline-directed medical therapies for acute HF (STRONG-HF) trial was published.[74] This study revealed that early and frequent outpatient visits for patients presenting with acute HF increased the likelihood of prescribing goal doses of HF GDMT compared to usual care and resulted in lower risk of combined death or future HF hospitalization. Although minoritized racial and ethnic groups were not well represented in this study, findings can still be extrapolated. In addition, standardized reminders for up titrating HF GDMT in the electronic medical record may help with clinical inertia as was observed in several single-center studies.[75,76]

Uninsurance and SDOH remain major barriers to appropriate HF care. Approaches to address these issues may warrant identifying community and institutional resources to allocate to patients

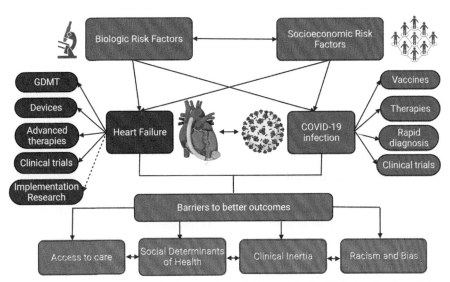

Fig. 1. The interplay between COVID-19 infection and heart failure. Biologic risk factors (such as diabetes, obesity, coronary disease, tobacco use, and so forth) combined with socioeconomic risk factors (such as inequalities in access to health care, education, wealth, high resource neighborhoods, and so forth) increase the risk of heart failure and COVID-19 infection. The rapid development of vaccines, therapies, and rapid diagnostic kits for COVID-19 as well as ongoing clinical trials has led to the resolution of the pandemic. A similar scenario has been seen in heart failure, where the use of guideline-directed medical therapy, implantable defibrillators, cardiac resynchronization therapy, left ventricular assist devices and cardiac transplantation have led to improvement in the mortality of this condition. However, unequitable delivery of treatment and care contribute to racial and ethnic disparities. Community-based participatory research and implementation science focused on strategies that address overlapping barriers may improve outcomes for both heart failure and COVID-19.

when needed.[77] At times technology such as telemedicine may be helpful to improve access to care, but investments aimed at narrowing the "digital divide" are needed.[78] Overall, health care systems must consider moving toward the routine assessment of SDOH followed by the management of SDOH. It has long been recognized that addressing SDOH are vital for improving health care disparities.[79–81] This line of research has been underfunded.[82,83] Additional support of studies that engage community-based participatory research and implementation science may finally lead to equity.

Bias and structural racism are principal drivers of health care disparities.[84] Therefore to achieve equity, concerted efforts are needed that cohere around eliminating structural racism from all facets of society. The agency for change is at the individual, corporate, community, health care systems, state, and national levels. Initiatives that actively promote diversity, equity, and inclusion (DEI) are an important tenet toward this end (eg, health care work force diversification, DEI in clinical trials and so forth).[85] Many strategies are structural (neighborhood and housing conditions for all people) or policy frameworks (eg, enacting of universal health care access), but some can be individual. Evidence-based bias reduction training has helped

enhance diverse hiring and selection of trainees as well as contribute to more equitable culture.[86,87] These same training courses may translate to better prescribing and allocation of therapies to minoritized racial and ethnic groups. In addition, a diverse and inclusive workforce may help reduce cardiovascular access disparities for patients with HF. For example, studies have reported that Black patients consistently experienced poorer communication quality, information-giving, patient participation, and participatory decision-making than White patients in studies examining the concordance of physician-patient interactions.[88]

SUMMARY

The COVID-19 pandemic highlighted existing inequities in HF care among minoritized racial and ethnic groups. Minoritized racial and ethnic groups had disproportionately worse cardiovascular outcomes during the pandemic including higher rates of death. The pandemic demonstrated the urgency to address clinical inertia, SDOH, bias, and structural racism. Equity in HF care may be achieved using strategies that bring about the standardization of optimal HF treatment, creatively address SDOH using community and institutional resources, and support systematic and individual changes to address structural racism and bias. Therefore, it is paramount to support research focused on strategies to correct disparities such as community-based participatory research and implementation science.

CLINICS CARE POINTS

- Develop clinic or system level resources to address social determinants of health.
- Identify clinic or system level policies that may systematically contribute to discrimination or racism in the care of population groups.
- Identify a patient's social determinants of health at each health encounter.
- Deploy resources to match patient needs.
- Iteratively assess relevant patient metrics to determine whether social determinants of health are being managed effectively.

FUNDING

This study was funded by Dr K. Breathett's research support from the National Heart, Lung, and Blood Institute, United States (NHLBI) K01HL142848, R56HL159216, R01HL159216, and L30HL148881.

REFERENCES

1. Betancourt JR, Maina AW. The Institute of Medicine report "Unequal Treatment": implications for academic health centers. Mt Sinai J Med 2004;71(5):314–21.
2. Williamson EJ, Walker AJ, Bhaskaran K, et al. Factors associated with COVID-19-related death using OpenSAFELY. Nature 2020;584(7821):430–6.
3. Ferdinand KC, Reddy TK. Disparities in the COVID-19 pandemic: a clarion call for preventive cardiology. Am J Prev Cardiol 2021;8:100283.
4. Goldman N, Andrasfay T. Life expectancy loss among Native Americans during the COVID-19 pandemic. Demogr Res Jul-Dec 2022;47:233–46.
5. Mwansa H, Lewsey S, Mazimba S, et al. Racial/ethnic and gender disparities in heart failure with reduced ejection fraction. Curr Heart Fail Rep 2021;18(2):41–51.
6. Tsao CW, Aday AW, Almarzooq ZI, et al. Heart disease and stroke statistics-2023 update: a report from the American heart association. Circulation 2023;147(8):e93–621.
7. Tsao CW, Aday AW, Almarzooq ZI, et al. Heart disease and stroke statistics-2022 update: a report from the American heart association. Circulation 2022;145(8):e153–639.
8. Writing Group M, Mozaffarian D, Benjamin EJ, et al. Executive summary: heart disease and stroke statistics–2016 update: a report from the American heart association. Circulation 2016;133(4):447–54.
9. Rodriguez CJ, Allison M, Daviglus ML, et al. Status of cardiovascular disease and stroke in Hispanics/Latinos in the United States: a science advisory from the American Heart Association. Circulation 2014;130(7):593–625.
10. Rangel MO, Kaplan R, Daviglus M, et al. Estimation of incident heart failure risk among US hispanics/latinos using a validated echocardiographic risk-stratification index: the echocardiographic study of latinos. J Card Fail 2018;24(9):622–4.
11. Breathett K, Sims M, Gross M, et al. Cardiovascular health in American Indians and Alaska natives: a scientific statement from the American heart association. Circulation 2020;141(25):e948–59.
12. Muller CJ, Noonan CJ, MacLehose RF, et al. Trends in cardiovascular disease morbidity and mortality in American Indians over 25 Years: the strong heart study. J Am Heart Assoc 2019;8(21):e012289.
13. Ilonze O, Free K, Breathett K. Unequitable heart failure therapy for black, hispanic and American-Indian patients. Card Fail Rev 2022;8:e25.
14. Ziaeian B, Kominski GF, Ong MK, et al. National differences in trends for heart failure hospitalizations by sex and race/ethnicity. Circ Cardiovasc Qual Outcomes 2017;10(7). https://doi.org/10.1161/CIRCOUTCOMES.116.003552.
15. Wadhera RK, Joynt Maddox KE, Wasfy JH, et al. Association of the hospital readmissions reduction program with mortality among medicare beneficiaries hospitalized for heart failure, acute myocardial infarction, and pneumonia. JAMA 2018;320(24):2542–52.
16. Hall ME, Vaduganathan M, Khan MS, et al. Reductions in heart failure hospitalizations during the COVID-19 pandemic. J Card Fail 2020;26(6):462–3.
17. Czeisler ME, Marynak K, Clarke KEN, et al. Delay or avoidance of medical care because of COVID-19-related concerns - United States, june 2020. MMWR Morb Mortal Wkly Rep 2020;69(36):1250–7.
18. Seervai S. The Dose. Want people to take the COVID-19 Vaccine? Confront Racism in Health Care. September 24th, 2021. https://www.commonwealthfund.org/publications/podcast/2021/sep/want-people-take-covid-19-vaccine-confront-racism-health-care.
19. Solomon KKaH. The Dangers of Confusing Vaccine Hesitancy with Vaccine Access. https://www.thinkglobalhealth.org/article/dangers-confusing-vaccine-hesitancy-vaccine-access.
20. Sahu KK, Mishra AK, Lal A. COVID-2019: update on epidemiology, disease spread and management. Monaldi Arch Chest Dis 2020;90(1). https://doi.org/10.4081/monaldi.2020.1292.
21. Breathett K. Health care equity cannot afford further delays. JACC Heart Fail 2021;9(10):720–1.

22. Zelner J, Trangucci R, Naraharisetti R, et al. Racial disparities in coronavirus disease 2019 (COVID-19) mortality are driven by unequal infection risks. Clin Infect Dis 2021;72(5):e88–95.

23. Khubchandani J, Macias Y. COVID-19 vaccination hesitancy in Hispanics and African-Americans: a review and recommendations for practice. Brain Behav Immun Health 2021;15:100277.

24. The Converdsation: Between Us, About Us, A New Campaign By Black Health Care Workers for Black People about the COVID-19 Vaccines. March 4th, 2021. https://www.greaterthancovid.org/the-conversation-between-us-about-us-a-new-campaign-by-black-health-care-workers-for-black-people-about-the-covid-19-vaccines/.

25. Prevention CfDCa. COVID-19 Vaccine Equity for Racial and Ethnic Minority Groups. Updated March 29th. https://www.cdc.gov/coronavirus/2019-ncov/community/health-equity/vaccine-equity.html.

26. Prevention CfDCa. Social Determinants of Health. Updated March 6th.

27. Whitman A. Addressing Social Determinants of Health: Examples of Successful Evidence-Based Strategies and Current Federal Efforts. 2022. Addressing Social Determinants of Health in Federal Programs.

28. Singu S, Acharya A, Challagundla K, et al. Impact of social determinants of health on the emerging COVID-19 pandemic in the United States. Front Public Health 2020;8:406.

29. Cajita MI, Cajita TR, Han HR. Health literacy and heart failure: a systematic review. J Cardiovasc Nurs 2016;31(2):121–30.

30. Fabbri M, Murad MH, Wennberg AM, et al. Health literacy and outcomes among patients with heart failure: a systematic review and meta-analysis. JACC Heart Fail 2020;8(6):451–60.

31. Lynch EE, Malcoe LH, Laurent SE, et al. The legacy of structural racism: associations between historic redlining, current mortgage lending, and health. SSM Popul Health 2021;14:100793.

32. Mujahid MS, Gao X, Tabb LP, et al. Historical redlining and cardiovascular health: the multi-ethnic study of atherosclerosis. Proc Natl Acad Sci U S A 2021;118(51). https://doi.org/10.1073/pnas.2110986118.

33. Rothstein R. The racial achievement gap, segregated schools, and segrated neighborhoods-A constitutional insult. Race and Social Problems 2015;7:21–30.

34. In: Smedley BD, Stith AY, Nelson AR, eds Unequal Treatment: Confronting Racial and Ethnic Disparities in Health Care. 2003.

35. Breathett K, Jones J, Lum HD, et al. Factors related to physician clinical decision-making for african-American and hispanic patients: a qualitative meta-synthesis. J Racial Ethn Health Disparities 2018;5(6):1215–29.

36. Sridhar AR, Yarlagadda V, Parasa S, et al. Cardiac resynchronization therapy: US trends and disparities in utilization and outcomes. Circ Arrhythm Electrophysiol 2016;9(3):e003108.

37. Farmer SA, Kirkpatrick JN, Heidenreich PA, et al. Ethnic and racial disparities in cardiac resynchronization therapy. Heart Rhythm 2009;6(3):325–31.

38. Zhang L, Sobolev M, Pina IL, et al. Predictors of cardiac rehabilitation initiation and adherence in a multiracial urban population. J Cardiopulm Rehabil Prev 2017;37(1):30–8.

39. Sun EY, Jadotte YT, Halperin W. Disparities in cardiac rehabilitation participation in the United States: a systematic review and META-analysis. J Cardiopulm Rehabil Prev 2017;37(1):2–10.

40. Li S, Fonarow GC, Mukamal K, et al. Sex and racial disparities in cardiac rehabilitation referral at hospital discharge and gaps in long-term mortality. J Am Heart Assoc 2018;7(8). https://doi.org/10.1161/JAHA.117.008088.

41. Breathett K, Allen LA, Helmkamp L, et al. The affordable care act medicaid expansion correlated with increased heart transplant listings in african-Americans but not hispanics or caucasians. JACC Heart Fail 2017;5(2):136–47.

42. Breathett KK, Xu H, Sweitzer NK, et al. Is the affordable care act medicaid expansion associated with receipt of heart failure guideline-directed medical therapy by race and ethnicity? Am Heart J 2022;244:135–48.

43. Breathett KK, Knapp SM, Wightman P, et al. Is the affordable care act medicaid expansion linked to change in rate of ventricular assist device implantation for blacks and whites? Circ Heart Fail 2020;13(4):e006544.

44. Mwansa H, Barry I, Knapp SM, et al. Association between the affordable care act medicaid expansion and receipt of cardiac resynchronization therapy by race and ethnicity. J Am Heart Assoc 2022;11(19):e026766.

45. Nayak A, Hicks AJ, Morris AA. Understanding the complexity of heart failure risk and treatment in black patients. Circ Heart Fail 2020;13(8):e007264.

46. Akwo EA, Kabagambe EK, Harrell FE Jr, et al. Neighborhood deprivation predicts heart failure risk in a low-income population of blacks and whites in the southeastern United States. Circ Cardiovasc Qual Outcomes 2018;11(1):e004052.

47. Shirey TE, Hu Y, Ko YA, et al. Relation of neighborhood disadvantage to heart failure symptoms and hospitalizations. Am J Cardiol 2021;140:83–90.

48. Gu SX, Tyagi T, Jain K, et al. Thrombocytopathy and endotheliopathy: crucial contributors to COVID-19 thromboinflammation. Nat Rev Cardiol 2021;18(3):194–209.

49. Writing C, Gluckman TJ, Bhave NM, et al. 2022 acc expert consensus decision pathway on cardiovascular

sequelae of COVID-19 in adults: myocarditis and other myocardial involvement, post-acute sequelae of SARS-CoV-2 infection, and return to play: a report of the American college of cardiology solution set oversight committee. J Am Coll Cardiol 2022;79(17): 1717–56.

50. Chen R, Lan Z, Ye J, et al. Cytokine storm: the primary determinant for the pathophysiological evolution of COVID-19 deterioration. Front Immunol 2021;12:589095.

51. Puntmann VO, Carerj ML, Wieters I, et al. Outcomes of cardiovascular magnetic resonance imaging in patients recently recovered from coronavirus disease 2019 (COVID-19). JAMA Cardiol 2020;5(11): 1265–73.

52. Jabri A, Kalra A, Kumar A, et al. Incidence of stress cardiomyopathy during the coronavirus disease 2019 pandemic. JAMA Netw Open 2020;3(7): e2014780.

53. Greene SJ, Lautsch D, Yang L, et al. Prognostic interplay between COVID-19 and heart failure with reduced ejection fraction. J Card Fail 2022;28(8): 1287–97.

54. Goyal P, Reshetnyak E, Khan S, et al. Clinical characteristics and outcomes of adults with a history of heart failure hospitalized for COVID-19. Circ Heart Fail 2021;14(9):e008354.

55. Salah HM, Fudim M, O'Neil ST, et al. Post-recovery COVID-19 and incident heart failure in the National COVID Cohort Collaborative (N3C) study. Nat Commun 2022;13(1):4117.

56. Babapoor-Farrokhran S, Alzubi J, Port Z, et al. Impact of COVID-19 on heart failure hospitalizations. SN Comprehensive Clinical Medicine 2021;3(10): 2088–92.

57. Shoaib A, Van Spall HGC, Wu J, et al. Substantial decline in hospital admissions for heart failure accompanied by increased community mortality during COVID-19 pandemic. European Heart Journal - Quality of Care and Clinical Outcomes 2021; 7(4):378–87.

58. Russo RG, Li Y, Đoàn LN, et al. COVID-19, social determinants of health, and opportunities for preventing cardiovascular disease: a conceptual framework. J Am Heart Assoc 2021;10(24):e022721.

59. Wadhera RK, Figueroa JF, Rodriguez F, et al. Racial and ethnic disparities in heart and cerebrovascular disease deaths during the COVID-19 pandemic in the United States. Circulation 2021;143(24):2346–54.

60. Janus SE, Makhlouf M, Chahine N, et al. Examining disparities and excess cardiovascular mortality before and during the COVID-19 pandemic. Mayo Clin Proc 2022.

61. Nunez A, Sreeganga SD, Ramaprasad A. Access to healthcare during COVID-19. Int J Environ Res Public Health 2021;18(6). https://doi.org/10.3390/ijerph18062980.

62. Giblin EM, Adams KF Jr, Hill L, et al. Comparison of hydralazine/nitrate and angiotensin receptor neprilysin inhibitor use among black versus nonblack Americans with heart failure and reduced ejection fraction (from CHAMP-HF). Am J Cardiol 2019; 124(12):1900–6.

63. Greene SJ, Butler J, Albert NM, et al. Medical therapy for heart failure with reduced ejection fraction: the CHAMP-HF registry. J Am Coll Cardiol 2018; 72(4):351–66.

64. Sandhu AT, Zheng J, Tisdale RL, et al. Medical therapy for patients with recent-onset heart failure with reduced ejection fraction during the COVID-19 pandemic: insights from the Veteran's affairs healthcare system. Am Heart J 2022;22:100210.

65. Yuan N, Botting PG, Elad Y, et al. Practice patterns and patient outcomes after widespread adoption of remote heart failure care. Circ Heart Fail 2021; 14(10):e008573.

66. Patel SY, Mehrotra A, Huskamp HA, et al. Variation in telemedicine use and outpatient care during the COVID-19 pandemic in the United States. Health Aff 2021;40(2):349–58.

67. Breathett K, Liu WG, Allen LA, et al. African Americans are less likely to receive care by a cardiologist during an intensive care unit admission for heart failure. JACC Heart Fail 2018;6(5):413–20.

68. Eberly LA, Richterman A, Beckett AG, et al. Identification of racial inequities in access to specialized inpatient heart failure care at an academic medical center. Circ Heart Fail 2019;12(11):e006214.

69. Colvin M, Smith JM, Ahn Y, et al. OPTN/SRTR 2020 annual data report: heart. Am J Transplant 2022; 22(Suppl 2):350–437.

70. Cascino TM, Colvin MM, Lanfear DE, et al. Racial inequities in access to ventricular assist device and transplant persist after consideration for preferences for care: a report from the revival study. Circ Heart Fail 2023;16(1):e009745.

71. Breathett K, Yee E, Pool N, et al. Does race influence decision making for advanced heart failure therapies? J Am Heart Assoc 2019;8(22):e013592.

72. Kahneman D. Thinking, fast and slow. New York City, NY: Farrar, Straus and Giroux; 2011. p. 499.

73. Rashid M, Timmis A, Kinnaird T, et al. Racial differences in management and outcomes of acute myocardial infarction during COVID-19 pandemic. Heart 2021;107(9):734–40.

74. Mebazaa A, Davison B, Chioncel O, et al. Safety, tolerability and efficacy of up-titration of guideline-directed medical therapies for acute heart failure (STRONG-HF): a multinational, open-label, randomised, trial. Lancet 2022;400(10367):1938–52.

75. Ghazi L, Yamamoto Y, Riello RJ, et al. Electronic alerts to improve heart failure therapy in outpatient practice: a cluster randomized trial. J Am Coll Cardiol 2022;79(22):2203–13.

76. Mukhopadhyay A, Reynolds HR, Phillips LM, et al. Cluster-randomized trial comparing ambulatory decision support tools to improve heart failure care. J Am Coll Cardiol 2023. https://doi.org/10.1016/j.jacc.2023.02.005.

77. Powell-Wiley TM, Baumer Y, Baah FO, et al. Social determinants of cardiovascular disease. Circ Res 2022;130(5):782–99.

78. Eberly LA, Khatana SAM, Nathan AS, et al. Telemedicine outpatient cardiovascular care during the COVID-19 pandemic: bridging or opening the digital divide? Circulation 2020;142(5):510–2.

79. Williams DR, Costa MV, Odunlami AO, et al. Moving upstream: how interventions that address the social determinants of health can improve health and reduce disparities. J Public Health Manag Pract 2008;14(Suppl):S8–17.

80. Breathett K, Spatz ES, Kramer DB, et al. The groundwater of racial and ethnic disparities research: a statement from circulation: cardiovascular quality and outcomes. Circ Cardiovasc Qual Outcomes 2021; 14(2):e007868.

81. Reopell L, Nolan TS, Gray DM 2nd, et al. Community engagement and clinical trial diversity: navigating barriers and co-designing solutions-A report from the "Health Equity through Diversity" seminar series. PLoS One 2023;18(2):e0281940.

82. Carnethon MR, Kershaw KN, Kandula NR. Disparities research, disparities researchers, and health equity. JAMA 2020;323(3):211–2.

83. Hoppe TA, Litovitz A, Willis KA, et al. Topic choice contributes to the lower rate of NIH awards to African-American/black scientists. Sci Adv 2019; 5(10):eaaw7238.

84. Churchwell K, Elkind MSV, Benjamin RM, et al. Call to action: structural racism as a fundamental driver of health disparities: a presidential advisory from the American heart association. Circulation 2020; 142(24):e454–68.

85. Williams DR, Cooper LA. Reducing racial inequities in health: using what we already know to take action. Int J Environ Res Public Health 2019;16(4). https://doi.org/10.3390/ijerph16040606.

86. Carnes M, Devine PG, Baier Manwell L, et al. The effect of an intervention to break the gender bias habit for faculty at one institution: a cluster randomized, controlled trial. Acad Med 2015;90(2):221–30.

87. Capers Qt, Clinchot D, McDougle L, et al. Implicit racial bias in medical school admissions. Acad Med 2017;92(3):365–9.

88. Sabin JA, Rivara FP, Greenwald AG. Physician implicit attitudes and stereotypes about race and quality of medical care. Med Care 2008;46(7):678–85.

The Economic Burden of Heart Failure with Reduced Ejection Fraction
Living Longer but Poorer?

Larry A. Allen, MD, MHS[a],*, Emily Fryman Lowe, MD[b],
Dan D. Matlock, MD, MPH[c]

KEYWORDS

• Heart failure • Cost and cost analysis • Health resources • Chronic disease • Financial stress

KEY POINTS

- HFrEF is typically a chronic and highly symptomatic disease, where multiple new treatments in recent years have been shown to improve survival but also add significant burdens and costs for patients.
- Understanding patient (and family caregiver) costs related to HFrEF management is critical to delivering patient-centered, high-value care that maximizes health outcomes and patient experience.
- Efforts to communicate and address health care costs are emerging, including tailored estimates of out-of-pocket costs for medications provided in real-time during clinical encounters.
- Given the significant costs to patients associated with the multiple medications and devices available for HFrEF, improving equitable access to care will require improved data on the relative value of treatments as well as changes in health care policy and financing.

CHRONIC DISEASES ARE COSTLY

Chronic diseases have significant health burdens and economic costs. Of the more than $4 trillion spent annually on health care in the United States (U.S.), 90% goes to people with chronic conditions.[1] When including the costs of lost economic productivity, chronic disease accounts for almost one-fifth of the American economy.[2,3] Significant advances in management have improved longevity and can increase the ability of afflicted individuals to remain functional, but overall have raised the burden of treatment. Polypharmacy, serial testing, and frequent encounters with the health care system are increasing. As are the costs of therapies, with newly approved drugs (including biologics) in the U.S. now priced at an average of more than $180,000 per year.[4]

Chronic health problems not only constitute a massive burden on the U.S. economy, but also come at the expense of individuals' physical and financial well-being. Cost and resource use are most often evaluated and reported from the perspective of payers (eg, Medicare) and society. Yet, understanding the patient perspective is of vital importance to the day-to-day experience of living with a chronic disease and in the individual medical decision making that determines actual care delivery and health outcomes (**Table 1**). Unfortunately, health care prices are neither simple nor transparent, such that patients and clinicians are often unable to easily assess costs.[5] With a

[a] Division of Cardiology, Department of Medicine, University of Colorado School of Medicine, 12631 East 17th Avenue, Academic Office One, #7019, Mailstop B130, Aurora, CO 80045, USA; [b] Department of Medicine, University of Colorado School of Medicine, 12631 East 17th Avenue, Mailstop B177, Aurora, CO 80045, USA; [c] Adult and Child Center for Outcomes Research and Delivery Science (ACCORDS), University of Colorado School of Medicine, Children's Hospital Colorado, 1890 North Revere Court, Mailstop F44, Aurora, CO 80045, USA
* Corresponding author.
E-mail address: larry.allen@cuanschutz.edu

Cardiol Clin 41 (2023) 501–510
https://doi.org/10.1016/j.ccl.2023.06.003

Table 1
Economic terms

Term	Perspective	Definition
Cost	Payers	The amount paid to providers for services rendered (typically a third-party health insurer).
	Providers	The expense incurred to deliver health care services to patients.
	Patients	The amount patients pay out-of-pocket for health care services (annual premiums and per service copays; lost wages or taxes are generally excluded from such calculations, despite their importance).
Charge or price	All	The amount asked by a health care provider (professional fee) or health system (facility fee) for a health care good or service, which appears on a medical bill.
Reimbursement or collection	All	A payment made by a third party to a provider for services. This may be an amount for every service delivered (fee-for-service), for each day in the hospital (per diem), for each episode of hospitalization (eg, diagnosis-related groups, or DRGs), or for each patient considered to be under their care (capitation). Patient copays may supplement third party payer reimbursement.

Adapted from Moriates C, Arora V, Shah N. Understanding Value-Based Healthcare. New York, NY: McGraw-Hill; 2015:27-28.

proliferation of high-deductible health plans in the U.S. and shift of health care costs to premiums and out-of-pocket (OOP) copays, direct health care payments by patients have increased. Concerns about out-of-pocket cost can influence patients' behavior and have been implicated in avoidance of medical care, nonadherence to medications, and the acceleration of health care disparities.[6] Medical debt is one of the most common causes of bankruptcy in the U.S.[7]

HEART FAILURE WITH REDUCED EJECTION FRACTION IS A PROTOTYPE FOR CHRONIC DISEASE

Heart failure with reduced ejection fraction (HFrEF) is an exemplar for the promise and peril of advances in chronic disease management. The lifetime risk of heart failure at 50 years of age among participants of the Framingham Heart Study (1990–2014) was 22.6% in females and 25.3% in males.[8] Of the more than 6 million Americans now living with chronic heart failure, approximately half have HFrEF. Heart failure has the highest projected increase in the prevalence of any cardiovascular disease in coming years, in part because it is most often a disease of aging. HFrEF is often the downstream result of other chronic conditions and persistent health behaviors—hypertension, diabetes, vascular disease,

obesity, smoking—such that the average patient with HFrEF has about 4.5 other chronic conditions,[9] which also demand chronic disease management.

Parallel to the rise in heart failure rates, the therapeutic armamentarium available for HFrEF has expanded. In the last decade, multiple new medications have been approved for use in patients with HFrEF, including the I_f inhibitor ivabradine, the angiotensin receptor-neprilysin inhibitor (ARNI) sacubitril/valsartan, sodium glucose like transporter-2 inhibitors (SGLT2i) dapagliflozin and empagliflozin, the soluble guanylate cyclase stimulator verigicuat, and new parenteral formulations of iron; all of these reduce morbidity and some improve survival.[10] Multiple medical devices are also available for HFrEF, including implantable cardioverter defibrillators (ICD), cardiac resynchronization therapy pacing (CRT), and mitral valve clipping; emerging devices include remote monitoring (eg, CardioMEMS), cardiac contractility modulation (CCM), and carotid baroreceptor stimulation (eg, Barostim); and durable left ventricular assist devices (LVAD).[10] Lastly, with the rising availability of suitable organ donors due to the use of hepatitis C virus positive donor, donation after circulatory death, as well as the opioid epidemic, the number of heart transplants performed annually has increased from ~2200 per year to ~4100 per year.[11] Meanwhile, the ability to evaluate and diagnose heart failure has also increased with the wider availability of cardiac imaging. In summary, there are a dizzying number of HFrEF care options.

The totality of these advances is impressive. Mortality declines have been attributed primarily to evidence-based approaches to treat HFrEF, including combination use of neurohormonal blockade.[12] Initiation of quadruple therapy—β-blockers, ARNI, mineralocorticoid receptor antagonists, and SGLT2i—is estimated to reduce the hazard ratio of cardiovascular death or heart failure hospitalization by more than double (HR, 0.38 [95% CI, 0.30–0.47]), resulting in an estimated 1.4 to 6.3 additional years alive.[13] However, these benefits of these therapies is typically additive, which also means that the cumulative burden of these advances is also significant.

HYPER-POLYPHARMACY

In adults aged ≥50 years with self-reported heart failure from the National Health and Nutrition Examination Survey (NHANES) 2003-2014, 26% of patients were prescribed 10 or more medications per day.[14] In another study of 2007–2014 Medicare claims data (Part A, Part B, and Part D) linked to electronic health records from 2 large networks in Boston, 2258 patients with HFrEF had 11.3 ± 5.7 of total filled prescriptions for distinct medications.[15] In the REGARDS study of patients hospitalized for heart failure, 84% at admission and 95% at discharge took ≥5 medications; and 42% at admission and 55% at discharge took ≥10 medications.[16] Hyper-polypharmacy (prescription of >10 medications) and its associated cost has become standard for the majority of patients with HFrEF.

SOCIETAL COSTS

With the increasing prevalence of HFrEF combined with treatments that tend to stabilize rather than cure disease, the overall cost of HFrEF continues to rise. From a societal perspective—i.e., a broad view of total opportunity costs regardless of who pays—total costs for heart failure in 2012 were estimated at $30.7 billion,[17] for which approximately half was attributable to HFrEF. Projections suggest that by 2030 the total cost of heart failure will increase to $69.8 billion, with new treatments concentrated in the HFrEF population.[17] Annual median heart failure-associated medical costs in the United States 2014-2020 were estimated at $24,383 per patient, with heart failure hospitalizations accounting for the majority ($15,879 per patient).[18]

Approximately two-thirds of direct medical costs are due to hospitalization. In the Nationwide Readmission Database, patients with a primary heart failure hospital admission between 2010 and 2014, the mean cost for patients without invasive care was $10,995 compared with $129,547 for receipt of circulatory support, $251,110 for LVAD implantation, and $293,575 for heart transplantation.[19] In addition to invasive procedures, the major contributors to inpatient heart failure care costs are comorbidities and subsequent readmissions.

PATIENT COSTS

Most patients have health insurance to cover the costs of health care. However, patients will often be required to pay a mix of fixed premiums (monthly), copayments (fixed small amount for a given service or a percentage of the charge), and the cost of uncovered services. Each health insurance product (of which there are thousands in the U.S.) may have different rules about patient coverage, copayments, deductibles, and maximums.

The amount that a patient may owe is further affected by the location of the good or service. For example, Medicare patients often pay a deductible of $1,260 for acute hospitalization, and then Medicare covers the rest up to 60 hospital days. But if a Medicare patient is seen in the emergency department and kept under "observation status," he or she is technically an outpatient, for which the copayment for hospital services may be as much as 20 percent of the total charge.[20] In recent years the use of observation status has increased, but to the financial detriment of some patients.

Despite some clinician reluctance to discuss cost as it relates to treatments with survival benefit, patients with HFrEF do want to know their costs so that they can use that to help guide their treatment decisions.[21] Some broad efforts at price transparency have been promoted over many decades, but to date they have been relatively limited in scope and effect.[22] At present, neither clinicians nor patients have out-of-pocket costs available at the time of clinical encounters in order to facilitate the integration of this information into decisions.

OUT-OF-POCKET MEDICATION COSTS

In contrast to off-patent medications with multiple generic options—beta blockers, ARB, MRA—that typically cost $4 or less per month, "cash" or "list" pricing for drugs still on-patent—including sacubitril-valsartan, SGLT2i, ivabradine, and vericiguat—each generally cost in excess of $500 for a 30-day prescription, exceeding $6,000 per year per drug. Therefore, the average patient requires some form of financial assistance (usually through health insurance) to reasonably access these drugs. For example, the average annualized OOP cost for patients with Medicare Part D coverage is $1685 for sacubitril/valsartan ($1400 more than the cost of an ARB alone)[23] and $1615 for dapagliflozin.[24] In a broader analysis using Optum data, monthly out-of-pocket (OOP) cost for sacubitril-valsartan, compared with angiotensin-converting enzyme inhibitors/angiotensin receptor blockers, was higher for both commercially insured patients (mean, $69 versus $6.74) and Medicare Advantage (mean, $62 versus $2.52).[25] For older patients with multiple chronic conditions including HFrEF, the average OOP cost of following guideline-directed medical therapy is substantial.[26]

However, estimating OOP patient costs for on-patent drugs can be quite challenging.[27] With thousands of insurance products, each with its own set of rules, clinicians cannot reasonably predict medication costs for individual patients. Furthermore, payments for many prescription drugs change over the course of a year based on cumulative OOP expenses as they relate to deductibles and OOP maximums.

An example of the complexity can be found in the stand-alone Medicare Part D prescription drug plan rules for 2023:[28]

- The subscriber pays a required, fixed monthly premium.
- The subscriber covers 100% of drug costs until they meet the $505 deductible.
- Upon meeting the deductible, subscribers enter the initial coverage phase where they must pay 25% of the cost of drugs until reaching total spending of $4,660.
- After the initial coverage period, the subscriber enters a coverage gap phase (ie, the "donut hole") wherein subscribers pay 25% for both brand-name and generic drugs, with manufacturers providing a 70% discount on brands and plans paying the remaining 5% of brand drug costs, and plans paying the remaining 75% of generic drug costs.
- When subscriber exceeds total drug costs of $11,206 for the year, they enter a catastrophic coverage phase, where Medicare pays 80%, plans pay 15%, and enrollees pay either 5% of total drug costs or $4.15/$10.35 for each generic and brand-name drug, respectively.

The U.S. federal government also establishes limits on how much a person or family will pay out of pocket annually under commercial insurance plans. Medicare Advantage (which has grown to nearly half of Medicare in recent years), and other "bundled" plans, are typically simpler in terms of copays. The Inflation Reduction Act of 2022 has further implications for drug costs and patient OOP spending[29]; rolling out over the next several years it has provisions that will address the lack of a hard cap on out-of-pocket spending for Part D enrollees, the inability of the federal government to negotiate drug prices with manufacturers, and drug pricing rising faster than the rate of inflation.

For commercial insurance plans, patient copays may be partially waived by the manufacturer for qualifying patients. For example, the manufacturers of sacubitril-valsartan provide a $10 copay card to eligible patients under commercial plans. Coupon or voucher offers by manufacturers are not allowed under Medicare. Other patient assistance programs exist, including means-tested provision of discounted or free medications to patients who are unable to afford them; however, these programs have limitations and administrative burdens. Help with navigating such patient assistant programs is available through nonprofit organizations.[30]

It will be some time before generic formulations of ivabradine, ARNIs, and SGLT2 inhibitors become available. Although ivabradine was eligible for patent challenges in April 2019, owing to patents and regulatory protections, its generic entry into the U.S. market is not likely to occur until after 2026. Similarly, sacubitril/valsartan was eligible for patent challenges in July 2019, but the earliest generic is not likely until after 2027. Dapagliflozin was eligible for patent challenges in January 2018, but is unlikely to have generic entry until after 2030. And empagliflozin's generic entry is estimated for 2034.[31]

CAREGIVER COSTS

The estimated value for the time caregivers of heart failure patients spend in their role has been estimated at $6.5 billion per year in the United States (2015 dollars) and is projected to increase to $13.5 billion per year by 2035.[32] Caregivers assume substantial OOP costs related to caregiving, often paired with irrecoverable loss of income, benefits, and career opportunities. These costs may be disproportionately borne by older adults, women, and minority populations already at higher risk for financial insecurity.[33]

INDIRECT COSTS

Indirect costs of a disease account for lost productivity including lost wages due to disability or death. The indirect costs of heart failure are estimated to increase from $10 billion in 2012 to $17 billion by 2030.[17]

Financial Toxicity

Because the average patient with HFrEF has more than 3 comorbid conditions and takes more than 10 medications, the cumulative treatment expenses can become overly burdensome. Financial toxicity is defined as "problems a patient has related to the cost of medical care."[34] In the Medical Expenditure Panel Survey 2014-2018, 858 had diagnoses of heart failure (representing 1.8 million patients annually) of whom 33% reported financial hardship due to medical bills, and 13.2% were not able to pay bills at all.[35] This underscores the importance of proactive management on the part of the clinician.

EFFORTS TO CONSIDER VALUE IN CLINICAL PRACTICE GUIDELINES AND POLICY RECOMMENDATIONS

Health care value is generally defined by the formula of outcomes over costs and has been proposed as a unifying approach to measure improvements in the quality and affordability of health care. Generally, we should prioritize treatments with high value first. However, value assessments can vary widely depending on (1) the outcome(s) chosen and (2) the cost perspective (ie, who is paying).[36] Nonetheless, crude estimates of value can help triage investments, coverage decisions, and medical decision making.

Britain's executive non-departmental National Institute for Health and Care Excellence (NICE) conducts evidence-based evaluations of the cost-effectiveness of new and existing medicines, treatments, and procedures.[37] It then publishes guidelines on their use of within the National Health Service for England and Wales. One aspect of these guidelines is the explicit determination of cost–benefit boundaries for certain technologies that it assesses.

The 2022 ACCF/AHA/HFSA Guidelines for Heart Failure specifically address cost.[10] Value statements were added for select recommendations when data from high-quality, cost-effectiveness studies were available. Dominant (cost saving) treatments for HFrEF include generic ACEi/ARB, beta-blockers, and MRAs. High-value interventions (costs per quality-adjusted life year [QALY] < $60,000) for HFrEF include ARNi, ICD, and CRT. Interventions of intermediate economic value (costs per QALY $60,000-$90,000) include SGLT2i, noting that a reduction in drug cost (through contract pricing, for example) would improve the cost per QALY and potentially make SGLT2i a high-value therapy, too. Transplantation, in appropriately selected patients, was also deemed of intermediate value. In contrast, although tafamidis garnered a Class or Recommendation 1, it was deemed to provide low economic value (>$180 000 per QALY gained) in patients with heart failure with wild-type or variant transthyretin cardiac amyloidosis (although, typically not HFrEF until end-stage disease). Similarly, durable LVAD was deemed to provide low to intermediate economic value based on current costs and outcomes. Therapies with uncertain benefit—e.g., wireless monitoring of the PA pressure by an implanted hemodynamic monitor—earned Class of Recommendation 2B and were deemed to provide uncertain value. How much these "value statements" will change practice remains to be seen, but the infusion of cost into care recommendations is an important change.

INTEGRATING PATIENT COST INTO MEDICAL DECISION MAKING

Although clinicians might sometimes prefer to avoid cost discussions with patients, health insurance coverage of medications and out-of-pocket costs are clearly relevant to patient experience and therefore must be addressed. Patients express a strong desire to have open and honest discussions with their clinicians about the costs of treatment.[21] However, discussing tradeoffs between cost and major outcomes such as mortality is relatively unfamiliar and complex. In reviewing 224 recorded cardiology encounters in which sacubitril-valsartan was discussed, only 40% included any discussion of cost; when cost was discussed, specific cost for that patient was almost never available.

Cost transparency appears to guide patient decisions. In a study in which patients with HFrEF were asked whether they would want to take sacubitril-valsartan if their doctor recommended it, 92% stated that they would take it at an incremental out-of-pocket cost of $5, while 43% would do so at an incremental out-of-pocket cost of $100.[38] In a similar online survey using Ipsos Knowledge Panel, in which 1013 people with a history of cardiac disease were randomly assigned to consider whether they would likely take sacubitril-valsartan at an out-of-pocket cost of $10, $50, and $100 per month, willingness was 85%, 61%, and 33%, respectively.[6] Income was associated with willingness to take the medication; however, out-of-pocket cost affected willingness to take the medication across all income categories.

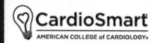

A DECISION AID FOR
RENIN-ANGIOTENSIN INHIBITOR DRUG OPTIONS FOR PATIENTS WITH HEART FAILURE

Including sacubitril/valsartan

▶ LET'S TALK COST

You may be wondering,
"How do I find out how much an ARNI will cost ME?"
There are two options to find out:

Option 1: Call your insurance company.
On the back of your insurance card, call the member services number and ask the representative the following:
"My clinician is considering prescribing the ARNI sacubitril/valsartan for me. Would you please tell me how much it would cost on my plan for a month of this medicine?" (60 tablets of 49/51 mg a month)

Option 2: Call your pharmacy.
Your clinician can begin a plan to switch you to an ARNI and write a prescription. You'll be able to see the cost before you finalize the plan, and decide whether you'd like to move forward. If you feel the cost is too high, you may leave the prescription unfilled; however, it's important you then get in touch with your clinician and work together to find a plan that will work better or you.

Write it down: An ARNI will cost **ME** per month: $ _____

Fig. 1. Patient decision aid on sacubitril/valsartan that focuses on patient costs. (*From* American College of Cardiology, CardioSmart. Drug Options for Patients With Heart Failure. https://www.cardiosmart.org/topics/heart-failure/assets/decision-aid/drug-options-for-patients-with-heart-failure Accessed February 27, 2023.)

All these data point toward the importance of providing cost in the context of clinical encounters to help facilitate more patient-centered decision-making. Moreover, the capacity to do so is growing. There are multiple integrated platforms being developed and implemented that can create tailored messaging, clinical decision support, and even populate patient-specific cost.

Fig. 2. Tailored estimates of patient out-of-pocket costs provided in the electronic health record provider order entry at the time of prescribing.[40]

▼ Prescriptions using OPTUM TEST PLAN (PBMNAME)

⊙ lisinopril (PRINIVIL,ZESTRIL) 20 mg tablet   💊 $0
    PATHSTONE HEALTH SER..., 30 tablet, 30 d
    Prior Authorization required

⊙ MIRAPEX ER 3.75 mg Tb24   💊 $747
    PATHSTONE HEALTH SER..., 30 tablet, 30 d $24.91/day
    Prior Authorization required

    Payer-Suggested Alternatives

    ○ PRAMIPEXOLE 3.75 mg Tb24   → $100
     PATHSTONE HEALTH... , 30 tablet, 30 d $3.34/day

⊙ metoprolol succinate (TOPROL-XL) 100 mg 24 hr ta... 💊 *Unknown*
    PATHSTONE HEALTH SER..., 90 tablet, 90 d
    Prior Authorization required. Drug not covered

Patient portion (per fill): $747

✓ Accept   ✗ Close

Your Heart Failure Medicines Checklist:
Work with your doctor for ONE Positive Change!

Below is a chart that shows the different heart failure medications. Please:
1) Check off <u>which medicines</u> you take in the "common names of medicine" column.
2) Fill in the <u>dose of medicine</u> that you take each day in the "my current dose" column.

Bring this chart to your next clinic appointment and discuss your medicines with your medical provider or doctor. **Aim to make one positive change.**

Medicine Family	Common Names of Medicine (Brand name)	My Current Dose	◎ Target Dose	Your Cost
Water Pill (diuretic)	☐ Furosemide (Lasix)		As much as you need to feel better	
	☐ Bumetanide (Bumex)			
	☐ Torsemide (Demadex)			
Adrenaline Blocking (beta blocker)	☐ Carvedilol (Coreg)		25–50 mg 2x per day	
	☐ Metoprolol Succinate (Toprol XL)		200 mg daily	
	☐ Bisoprolol (Zebeta)		10 mg daily	
Blood Vessel Relaxing (ACE/ARB)	☐ Sacubutril/Valsartan (Entresto) [recommended medicine]		97/103 mg 2x per day	
	☐ Lisinopril (Prinivil or Zestril)		20–40 mg daily	
	☐ Enalapril (Vasotec)		10–20 mg 2x per day	
	☐ Captopril (Capoten)		50 mg 2x per day	
	☐ Ramipril (Altace)		10 mg daily	
	☐ Losartan (Cozaar)		100–150 mg daily	
	☐ Candesartan (Atacand)		32 mg daily	
	☐ Valsartan (Diovan)		160 mg 2x per day	
Potassium Raising	☐ Spironolactone (Aldactone)		50 mg daily	
	☐ Eplerenone (Inspra)		50 mg daily	
Sodium Glucose Eliminating	☐ Canagliflozin (Invokana)		100 mg daily	
	☐ Dapagliflozin (Farxiga)		10 mg daily	
	☐ Empagliflozin (Jardiance)		10 mg daily	
	☐ Ertugliflozin (Steglatro)		5 mg or 15 mg daily	
OTHERS to consider	☐ Hydralazine/Isosorbide		100 mg/40 mg 3x per day	
	☐ Ivabradine (Corlanor)		7.5 mg 2x per day	
	☐ Digoxin (Lanoxin or Digoxin)		Depends on kidney function (0.0625-0.25 mg daily or every other day)	

Remember: **YOU** are the person who knows you best. **YOU** have the most to gain by being on the best treatments possible. **YOU** have a right to ask questions about your own care!

Fig. 3. Comprehensive HFrEF medication options, with the goal in including tailored out-of-pocket costs for all available options all at once to facilitate improved shared decision making inclusive of costs.[41,42]

To help patients anticipate out-of-pocket costs for HFrEF medications, the ACC partnered with the Colorado Program for Patient-Centered Decisions develop a patient decision aid for renin-angiotensin inhibitor drug options for patients with heart failure.[21] Two pages of this four-page decision aid are dedicated to helping patients obtain estimated out-of-pocket costs for sacubitril-valsartan because that is the main risk burden of this drug. The decision aid suggests two options to help patients find out what portion of drug cost they will be responsible for based on their insurance coverage—contacting their insurer or having the prescription for the drug run through the pharmacy (**Fig. 1**).[39]

Greater interoperability of electronic health records with insurers' databases has begun to enable real-time estimates of out-of-pocket costs provided at the time an electronic prescription is written. Electronic health record software vendors and health systems have worked to integrate estimate OOP costs into the flow of care. Real-time estimates are specific to patient insurance and selected pharmacy, orchestrated through a third-party vendor (**Fig. 2**).[40] Such functionality is not currently widely available, but is likely to become more so in the future.

While estimating OOP cost in the encounter at the time a prescription is written is an improvement, it is still too far downstream to optimally guide medical decision-making: i.e., cost is provided after a decision to prescribe is made. More relevant to actual medical decision making would be the provision of all OOP costs for relevant treatment options that are being considered, so that medical decision making is integrative. For example, in a patient with stable HFrEF, normal vitals, and renal function, who is on metoprolol succinate 200 mg PO daily, losartan 100 mg daily, and spironolactone 25 mg daily, a relevant discussion in the clinic would potentially include switching from ARB to ARNI and/or addition of SGLT2i. Having patient-specific estimated OOP cost available for sacubitril/valsartan, dapagliflozin, and empagliflozin all at the same time is likely to facilitate optimal shared decision making (**Fig. 3**).[41,42]

HEALTH POLICY AND PAYMENT

Despite the advancement in treatment options available for patients with HFrEF, the overall quality of care for HFrEF varies greatly across the United States. A major obstacle in trying to improve the quality of care is the current payment system, which is mostly a fee-for-service reimbursement system.[43] Rewarding volume has promoted fragmented and low-value care. Recognizing the need for change, the Centers for Medicare and Medicaid Services (CMS) Innovation Center created a new vision or "Strategy Refresh," with the goal of achieving equitable outcomes through high-quality, affordable, and patient-centered care through 5 objectives–Drive accountable care, advance health equity, support care innovations, improve access by addressing affordability, partner to achieve system transformation.[44] The American Heart Association and Duke Margolis Health Policy Center collaborated to provide cardiovascular health specific recommendations for each CMS objective to create a Value-Based Payment model for heart health.[43] Adopting such a new payment system promises to improve the quality of care for patients with cardiovascular disease by providing patient-centered, affordable, team-based comprehensive care.

SUMMARY

In summary, HFrEF is a chronic disease typically associated with aging, multimorbidity, progressive symptoms, and reduced survival. Patients with HFrEF have benefitted from a proliferation of treatments in recent years. But this increasing complexity of care options has also added significant burdens and costs relevant to payers, providers, and patients. Concerns about patient out-of-pocket cost have been implicated in avoidance of medical care, nonadherence to medications, and the exacerbation of health care disparities. Understanding patient (and caregiver) costs related to HFrEF is critical to delivering patient-centered, high-value care that maximizes health outcomes. Efforts to communicated and address health care costs are emerging, including tailored, real-time provision of OOP costs during encounters that can guide medical decision making. Ultimately equitable access to HFrEF care will require improved data on value and major changes in health care policy and financing.

CLINICS CARE POINTS

- Hyper-polypharmacy has become the standard for most patients living with HFrEF. Therefore completing a thorough medication reconciliation, and practicing shared decision making with the patient can significantly cut down on patient out of pocket cost and overall financial burden of living with a chronic disease such as HFrEF.

- Engage in cost discussions with patients regarding health insurance coverage and out-of-pocket costs related to HFrEF treatment to truly maximize patient experience and health outcomes. Refer to the 2022 ACCF/AHA/HFSA Guidelines for Heart Failure that specifically address cost when discussing with patients' treatment options.
- Cost transparency has been shown to guide patient decisions highlighting the importance of having access to cost during a clinical encounter. Use tools to help patients anticipate out-of-pocket costs for HFrEF medications.

DISCLOSURES

Dr L.A. Allen has received grant funding from NIH, United States and PCORI; and consulting fees from ACI Clinical, American Heart Association, Boston Scientific, Cytokinetics, Novartis, Quidel, StoryHealth, and UpToDate. Drs D.D. Matlock and E. Lowe have nothing to disclose.

REFERENCES

1. Health and Economic Costs of Chronic Diseases, National Center for Chronic Disease Prevention and Health Promotion (NCCDPHP), Centers for Disease Control and Prevention. Available at: https://www.cdc.gov/chronicdisease/about/costs/index.htm. Accessed February 27, 2023.
2. Buttorff C, Ruder T, Bauman M. Multiple chronic conditions in the United States. Santa Monica, CA: Rand Corp.; 2017. Available at: https://www.rand.org/pubs/tools/TL221.html. Accessed February 27, 2023.
3. National Health Expenditure Data: Historical. Center for Medicare & Medicaid Services. December 15, 2021. Available at: https://www.cms.gov/Research-Statistics-Data-and-Systems/Statistics-Trends-and-Reports/NationalHealthExpendData/NationalHealth AccountsHistorical. Accessed February 27, 2023.
4. Rome BN, Egilman AC, Kesselheim AS. Trends in prescription drug launch prices, 2008-2021. JAMA 2022;327(21):2145–7.
5. Arora V, Moriates C, Shah N. The challenge of understanding health care costs and charges. AMA J Ethics 2015;17(11):1046–52.
6. Rao BR, Speight CD, Allen LA, et al. Impact of financial considerations on willingness to take sacubitril/valsartan for heart failure. J Am Heart Assoc 2022; 11(12):e023789.
7. Himmelstein DU, Lawless RM, Thorne D, et al. Medical bankruptcy: still common despite the affordable care act. Am J Public Health 2019;109(3):431–3.
8. Tsao CW, Aday AW, Almarzooq ZI, et al. American heart association council on epidemiology and prevention statistics committee and stroke statistics subcommittee. Heart disease and stroke statistics-2023 update: a report from the American heart association. Circulation 2023;147(8):e93–621. Epub 2023 Jan 25. [Erratum in: Circulation. 2023 Feb 21; 147(8):e622]. PMID: 36695182.
9. Saczynski JS, Go AS, Magid DJ, et al. Patterns of comorbidity in older adults with heart failure: the Cardiovascular Research Network PRESERVE study. J Am Geriatr Soc 2013;61(1):26–33.
10. Heidenreich PA, Bozkurt B, Aguilar D, et al. 2022 AHA/ACC/HFSA guideline for the management of heart failure: executive summary: a report of the American college of cardiology/American heart association joint committee on clinical practice guidelines. Circulation 2022;145(18):e876–94.
11. United Network for Organ Sharing. Available at: https://unos.org/data/. Accessed February 27, 2023.
12. Merlo M, Pivetta A, Pinamonti B, et al. Long-term prognostic impact of therapeutic strategies in patients with idiopathic dilated cardiomyopathy: changing mortality over the last 30 years. Eur J Heart Fail 2014;16(3):317–24.
13. Vaduganathan M, Claggett BL, Jhund PS, et al. Estimating lifetime benefits of comprehensive disease-modifying pharmacological therapies in patients with heart failure with reduced ejection fraction: a comparative analysis of three randomised controlled trials. Lancet 2020;396(10244):121–8.
14. Kennel PJ, Kneifati-Hayek J, Bryan J, et al. Prevalence and determinants of hyperpolypharmacy in adults with heart failure: an observational study from the national health and nutrition examination survey (NHANES). BMC Cardiovasc Disord 2019; 19(1):76.
15. Umarje S, Vaduganathan M, Levin R, et al. Medication burden in older patients with heart failure: a cohort study of medicare beneficiaries. J Card Fail 2020;26(8):742–4.
16. Unlu O, Levitan EB, Reshetnyak E, et al. Polypharmacy in older adults hospitalized for heart failure. Circ Heart Fail 2020;13(11):e006977.
17. Heidenreich PA, Albert NM, Allen LA, et al. American heart association advocacy coordinating committee; council on arteriosclerosis, thrombosis and vascular biology; council on cardiovascular radiology and intervention; council on clinical cardiology; council on epidemiology and prevention; stroke council. Forecasting the impact of heart failure in the United States: a policy statement from the American Heart Association. Circ Heart Fail 2013;6(3):606–19.
18. Urbich M, Globe G, Pantiri K, et al. A systematic review of medical costs associated with heart failure in the USA (2014-2020). Pharmacoeconomics 2020; 38(11):1219–36.

19. Kwok CS, Abramov D, Parwani P, et al. Cost of inpatient heart failure care and 30-day readmissions in the United States. Int J Cardiol 2021;329:115–22.

20. Sheehy AM, Graf BK, Gangireddy S, et al. "Observation status" for hospitalized patients: implications of a proposed Medicare rules change. JAMA Intern Med 2013;173(21):2004–6.

21. Venechuk GE, Allen LA, Doermann Byrd K, et al. Conflicting perspectives on the value of neprilysin inhibition in heart failure revealed during development of a decision aid focusing on patient costs for sacubitril/valsartan. Circ Cardiovasc Qual Outcomes 2020;13(9):e006255.

22. Parente ST. Estimating the impact of new health price transparency policies. Inquiry 2023;60. https://doi.org/10.1177/00469580231155988. 469580231155988.

23. DeJong C, Kazi DS, Dudley RA, et al. Assessment of national coverage and out-of-pocket costs for sacubitril/valsartan under medicare part D. JAMA Cardiol 2019;4(8):828–30.

24. DeJong C, Masuda C, Chen R, et al. Out-of-pocket costs for novel guideline-directed diabetes therapies under medicare part D. JAMA Intern Med 2020;180(12):1696–9.

25. Shore S, Basu T, Kamdar N, et al. Use and out-of-pocket cost of sacubitril-valsartan in patients with heart failure. J Am Heart Assoc 2022;11(17):e023950.

26. Zhou T, Liu P, Dhruva SS, et al. Assessment of hypothetical out-of-pocket costs of guideline-recommended medications for the treatment of older adults with multiple chronic conditions, 2009 and 2019. JAMA Intern Med 2022;182(2):185–95.

27. Allen LA, Sarni SJ. Tips for Navigating Prior Authorization and Out-of-Pocket Costs for HFrEF Medications. Available at: https://www.medscape.com/viewarticle/950209_4. Accessed February 27, 2023.

28. Kaiser Family Foundation. An Overview of the Medicare Part D Prescription Drug Benefit. Available at: https://www.kff.org/medicare/fact-sheet/an-overview-of-the-medicare-part-d-prescription-drug-benefit/. Accessed February 27, 2023.

29. Kaiser Family Foundation. How Will the Prescription Drug Provisions in the Inflation Reduction Act Affect Medicare Beneficiaries? Available at:https://www.kff.org/medicare/issue-brief/how-will-the-prescription-drug-provisions-in-the-inflation-reduction-act-affect-medicare-beneficiaries/. Accessed February 27, 2023.

30. NeedyMeds. Available at: https://www.needymeds.org/. Accessed February 27, 2023.

31. DrugPatentWatch. Available at: https://www.drugpatentwatch.com/p/tradename/jardiance. Accessed February 27, 2023.

32. Dunbar SB, Khavjou OA, Bakas T, et al. American heart association. projected costs of informal caregiving for cardiovascular disease: 2015 to 2035: a policy statement from the American heart association. Circulation 2018;137(19):e558–77.

33. Kitko L, McIlvennan CK, Bidwell JT, et al. American heart association council on cardiovascular and stroke nursing; council on quality of care and outcomes research; council on clinical cardiology; and council on lifestyle and cardiometabolic health. family caregiving for individuals with heart failure: a scientific statement from the American heart association. Circulation 2020;141(22):e864–78.

34. Definition of fincial toxicity. National Cancer Institute. Available at: https://www.cancer.gov/publications/dictionaries/cancer-terms/def/financial-toxicity. Accessed February 27, 2023.

35. Ali HR, Valero-Elizondo J, Wang SY, et al. Subjective financial hardship due to medical bills among patients with heart failure in the United States: the 2014-2018 medical expenditure panel survey. J Card Fail 2022;28(9):1424–33.

36. Kini V, Michael Ho P. Toward patient-centered healthcare value. Circ Cardiovasc Qual Outcomes 2019;12(5):e005801.

37. National Institute for Health and Care Excellence. Available at: https://www.nice.org.uk/. Accessed February 27, 2023.

38. Smith GH, Shore S, Allen LA, et al. Discussing out-of-pocket costs with patients: shared decision making for sacubitril-valsartan in heart failure. J Am Heart Assoc 2019;8(1):e010635.

39. American College of Cardiology, CardioSmart. Drug Options for Patients With Heart Failure. Available at: https://www.cardiosmart.org/topics/heart-failure/assets/decision-aid/drug-options-for-patients-with-heart-failure. Accessed February 27, 2023.

40. TailorMed. Available at: https://tailormed.co/. Accessed February 27, 2023.

41. Allen LA, Venechuk G, McIlvennan CK, et al. An electronically delivered patient-activation tool for intensification of medications for chronic heart failure with reduced ejection fraction: the EPIC-HF trial. Circulation 2021;143(5):427–37.

42. The EPIC-HF medication checklist. Available at: https://patientdecisionaid.org/heart-failure-medication-epic/. Accessed February 27, 2023.

43. Churchwell K, Lloyd-Jones DM, Phelps M. Shaping value-based payment policy: improving heart health through value-based payment. Circulation 2022;145(11):e765–7. Erratum in: Circulation. 2022 Apr 5;145(14):e806. PMID: 35286169.

44. Centers for Medicare and Medicaid Services. Innovation Center Strategy Refresh. Available at: https://innovation.cms.gov/strategic-direction-whitepaper. Accessed February 27, 2023.

Sequencing Quadruple Therapy for Heart Failure with Reduced Ejection Fraction: Does It Really Matter?

Jiun-Ruey Hu, MD, MPH[a], Alexandra N. Schwann, MD[b], Jia Wei Tan, MD[c], Abdulelah Nuqali, MBBS[a], Ralph J. Riello, PharmD[a], Michael H. Beasley, MD[a,*]

KEYWORDS

- Guideline-directed medical therapy • Heart failure with reduced ejection fraction • Tolerability
- Sequence • Renin–angiotensin aldosterone system inhibitors • Beta blockers
- Mineralocorticoid receptor antagonists • Sodium–glucose cotransporter 2 inhibitors

KEY POINTS

- The conventional sequence of guideline-directed medical therapy (GDMT) initiation (renin–angiotensin system inhibitors- > beta blockers- > mineralocorticoid receptor antagonists [MRAs]- > sodium–glucose cotransporter 2 inhibitors [SGLT2i]) assumes that the effectiveness and tolerability of GDMT agents mirror the order in which they were historically developed, which is not true.
- Flexible GDMT sequencing should be permitted in special populations, such as patients with low blood pressure, low heart rate, chronic kidney disease, or atrial fibrillation.
- The initiation of certain GDMT medications may enable or increase tolerance of other GDMT medications (eg, SGLT2i reducing the risk of hyperkalemia and worsening renal function, thus enabling the use of angiotensin and neprilysin inhibitors and MRA), so sequencing strategy plays a role in at-risk populations.
- The achievement of partial doses of all four pillars of GDMT is better than achievement of full doses of incomplete (< four) pillars of GDMT.
- Deferring initiation of GDMT to the outpatient setting carries a greater than 75% chance that it will not be started within the next year due to therapeutic inertia and the "stickiness" of medications carried over from the inpatient setting.

INTRODUCTION

Although the development of novel pharmacologic treatments, interventional techniques, and advanced therapies for patients with heart failure (HF) has ushered in a mini-renaissance for the management of after decades of stagnancy, the implementation of guideline-directed medical therapy (GDMT) remains the bedrock of HF treatment. The primary goal of clinicians caring for patients with HF with reduced ejection fraction (HFrEF) is to prolong high-quality life with the fewest invasive interventions possible. This is the promise of GDMT. Patients with new onset HF

[a] Clinical and Translational Research Accelerator, Yale School of Medicine, New Haven, CT 06520, USA; [b] Department of Internal Medicine, Yale New Haven Hospital, P.O. Box 208030, New Haven, CT, 06520-8030, USA; [c] Division of Nephrology, Stanford University School of Medicine, 780 Welch Road, Palo Alto, CA 94304, USA
* Corresponding author.
E-mail address: michael.beasley@yale.edu
Twitter: @ruey_hu (J.-R.H.); @aschwann212 (A.N.S.); @jiiiiawei (J.W.T.); @AbdulelahNuqali (A.N.); @ralphadelta (R.J.R.); @MHBeasleyMD (M.H.B.)

Cardiol Clin 41 (2023) 511–524
https://doi.org/10.1016/j.ccl.2023.06.007

may initially present in cardiogenic shock. Yet after hemodynamic stabilization, initiation of GDMT, close monitoring, and outpatient follow-up, it is not uncommon for systolic function to markedly improve, allowing the patient to return to normal life. This return to normalcy can persist for many years, as long as disease-modifying therapies are continued.[1] How should clinicians implement these life-saving treatments for patients with HFrEF? Does the sequence in which GDMT matter as long as all recommended classes of therapy are eventually prescribed?

In practice, there may be as many methods of initiating and titrating as there are cardiologists. The latest American College of Cardiology/American Heart Association/Heart Failure Society of America guidelines strongly recommend early initiation of all four pillars of GDMT: (1) renin–angiotensin system inhibitors (RAASis) including angiotensin-converting enzyme inhibitors (ACEis)/angiotensin receptor blockers (ARBs)/angiotensin and neprilysin inhibitors (ARNis), (2) beta blockers (BBs), (3) mineralocorticoid receptor antagonists (MRAs), and (4) sodium–glucose cotransporter 2 inhibitors (SGLT2is) for patients with HFrEF.[2] Further details can be found at www.GDMT.org.[3] We recognize the importance of broad implementation of all four classes of GDMT as soon as possible, followed by rapid titration (**Table 1**) to target or maximally tolerated dosing. The purpose of this review is to highlight certain clinical scenarios in which the order of GDMT initiation during an acute HF (AHF) hospitalization can play a significant role.

TOLERABILITY, SAFETY, AND EFFICACY

Inpatient initiation and intensive up-titration of GDMT for patients hospitalized with AHF was examined in the STRONG-HF trial.[4] It compared a high-intensity intervention involving the rapid up-titration of GDMT versus usual care among patients with an admission for AHF. Intensive GDMT implementation and close follow-up was not only safe but also reduced the risk of 180-day all-cause mortality or HF readmission by 34%, with an adjusted risk difference of 8.1% ($P = .0021$) and adjusted risk ratio of 0.66.[4] The study was terminated early due to a larger than expected risk reduction of the primary endpoint in the high-intensity care group. Of note, patients were enrolled in this trial before the approval of SGLT2i for HFrEF. Thus, the GDMT in this study included ACEi/ARB/ARNi, BB, and MRA.

RENIN–ANGIOTENSIN SYSTEM INHIBITORS

Traditionally, patients with HFrEF were prescribed an ACEi or ARB as foundational disease-modifying therapy. Given the superior morbidity and mortality reduction seen with ARNi, sacubitril–valsartan is now the preferred RAASi—even in *de novo* HFrEF. It is also strongly recommended to actively transition stable patients on an ACEi or ARB to an ARNI as soon as possible.[5] Inpatient initiation of ARNI in patients with *de novo* HFrEF is supported by the PIONEER-HF trial.[6] In this study, 881 patients with HFrEF hospitalized for AHF were randomized to sacubitril–valsartan or enalapril after hemodynamic stabilization, defined as the absence of intravenous (IV) inotropic medication within 24 hours and no IV vasodilators, diuretic dose escalation, or systolic blood pressure of less than 100 mm Hg in the previous 6 hours. Patients initiated on sacubitril–valsartan had significantly lower N-terminal pro-B-type natriuretic peptide (NT-proBNP) serum concentrations at 8 weeks (−46.7% vs −25.3%, $P<.001$). Of note, the rates of worsening renal function (WRF), hyperkalemia, and symptomatic hypotension were similar between the treatment groups, supporting the safety and tolerability of in-hospital ARNi initiation. This study also highlights the potential benefit of sacubitril–valsartan in an expansive cohort of American patients, including decompensated patients with a history of HF and those with newly diagnosed HF.

BETA BLOCKERS

In patients hospitalized with AHF, the initiation of BB therapy is often delayed due to concerns that sympathetic nervous system antagonism may exacerbate an acute decompensation—particularly if incorporated before decongestion and hemodynamic stability. It is important for providers to recognize low-output states and cardiogenic shock early as BB should indeed be avoided during this period. In the appropriate hospitalized HF population, however, BB treatment before discharge is associated with improved clinical outcomes. IMPACT-HF randomized 375 patients admitted with AHF to either in-hospital carvedilol introduction before discharge or delayed carvedilol initiation at least 2 weeks after discharge during routine outpatient follow-up. Patients treated with carvedilol in the acute care setting—approximately 60 hours into hospital admission—had significantly better medication adherence (91.2% vs 73.4%, $P<.0001$) and a greater likelihood of reaching target dosing within 60 days. Inpatient initiation of carvedilol did not seem to confer any increased risk for adverse events including similar length of stay, rates of worsening HF, hypotension, or bradycardia.[7] BBs are commonly reported to have adverse effects, including dizziness, bradycardia, and low blood pressure, and these may

Table 1
Examples of studies that involved initiation or up-titration of guideline-directed medical therapy in patients hospitalized with heart failure

Class	Target Dose	Adverse Effects	Monitoring Parameters	NNT for All-Cause Mortality[2] (Standardized to 36 mo)
β-Blocker	• Bisoprolol 10 mg daily • Carvedilol 25 mg BID, if < 85kg • Carvedilol 50 mg BID, if ≥ 85 kg • Metoprolol Succinate 200 mg daily	• Bradycardia • Dizziness • Fatigue • Hypotension	• Blood pressure • Heart rate	9
ACEi	• Captopril 50 mg 3× daily • Enalapril 10–20 mg BID • Lisinopril 20–40 mg daily • Ramipril 10 mg daily • Trandolapril 4 mg daily	• Acute kidney injury • Angioedema • Cough • Hyperkalemia • Hypotension	• Blood pressure • Potassium • Serum creatinine	26
ARB	• Candesartan 32 mg daily • Losartan 150 mg daily • Valsartan 160 mg BID	• Acute kidney injury • Hyperkalemia • Hypotension	• Blood pressure • Potassium • Serum creatinine	26
ARNi	Sacubitril–valsartan 97–103 mg BID	• Acute kidney injury • Angioedema • Cough • Hyperkalemia • Hypotension	• Blood pressure • Potassium • NT-proBNP • Serum creatinine	27
MRA	• Eplerenone 50 mg daily • Spironolactone 50 mg daily	• Hyperkalemia • Gynecomastia (S > E)	• Blood pressure • Potassium • Serum creatinine	6
SGLT2i	• Dapagliflozin 10 mg daily • Empagliflozin 10 mg daily	• Acute kidney injury • Dyslipidemia • Genital mycotic infection • Hypoglycemia • Ketoacidosis • Urinary tract infection	• Glucose • Hemoglobin A1c • Serum creatinine • Volume status	22

Abbreviations: ACEi, angiotensin converting enzyme inhibitor; ARB, angiotensin receptor blocker; ARNi, angiotensin receptor-neprilysin inhibitor; MRA, mineralocorticoid receptor antagonist; NT-proBNP, N-terminal proB-type natriuretic peptide; SGLT2i, sodium–glucose cotransporter 2 inhibitor.

lead to intolerance and discontinuation with chronic treatment.[8] Given the significant mortality benefit in patients receiving all four classes of GDMT, clinicians can consider low dosing and slow up-titration of BB to better improve tolerability. It should be noted that although the practice of initiating metoprolol tartrate with transition to metoprolol succinate is prevalent in AHF, this is a practice likely carried over from acute myocardial infarction management and is not supported by clinical trial evidence in HFrEF.

MINERALOCORTICOID RECEPTOR ANTAGONISTS

Despite the immense magnitude of mortality benefit and long-standing affordability, MRA is the least frequently prescribed pillar of GDMT.[9] Concerns limiting prescriber uptake of MRA include the perceived risk of hyperkalemia or WRF.[10] The COACH trial found reduced 30-day mortality and rehospitalization rate in patients admitted with AHF who were discharged on spironolactone, with more notable benefit in higher risk patients, compared with patients not discharged on spironolactone (hazard ratio [HR] 0.362, $P = .027$).[11] The ATHENA-HF trial randomized MRA naive or low-dose MRA patients who presented with at least one sign or symptom of HF with concurrent elevation in NT-proBNP greater than 1000 pg/mL within 24 hours of admission to spironolactone or placebo. Although MRA treatment did not demonstrate improvement in the primary or secondary outcomes, high-dose spironolactone was shown to be well tolerated in the hospital setting without any increased risk of hyperkalemia or decreased renal function when compared with placebo.[12] To decrease the risk of hyperkalemia, the initiation of potassium binding resins and/or consideration of MRA dose reductions or alternate day dosing should be considered before discontinuation of therapy.[13,14] Hyperkalemia risk among MRAs may be related to differences in mineralocorticoid receptor selectivity and relative concentrations in cardiac versus renal tissues; there is some evidence to suggest that spironolactone may carry a higher risk of hyperkalemia, however, there has never been a direct comparison between the two drugs.[15] Eplerenone generally confers fewer adverse drug effects than spironolactone, most notably for gynecomastia and other sexual side effects which are known to be a reason for nonadherence among patients.[16] Initiation and continuation of MRA therapy can be challenging in certain patient populations, as its use is contraindicated in men with a serum creatinine greater than 2.5 mg/dL and women with a serum creatinine greater than 2mg/dL as well as all patients with an estimated glomerular filtration rate (eGFR) $\leq$ 30mL/min/1.73m.[2]

SODIUM–GLUCOSE COTRANSPORTER 2 INHIBITORS

SGLT2i are the newest pillar of GDMT. Initially approved for the treatment of type 2 diabetes mellitus, the significant morbidity and mortality benefit of this class is noted to be independent of whether a patient is diabetic or not. Unlike other classes of GDMT, SGLT2i are the simplest to add to a patient's regimen given their tolerability and once daily dosing with no need for titration. The EMPULSE trial randomized 530 patients admitted for AHF to empagliflozin or placebo and found a reduced risk of all-cause mortality and HF events at 90 days in the patients randomized to empagliflozin. Patients in the empagliflozin arm were also found to have improvement in their HF symptoms.[17] A meta-analysis of the DAPA-HF and EMPEROR-Reduced trials noted that empagliflozin and dapagliflozin were associated with a reduction in all-cause death, cardiovascular death, and rate of HF hospitalization with improved renal outcomes.[18] The EMPA-RESPONSE-AHF randomized 80 diabetic and nondiabetic patients admitted with AHF to empagliflozin or placebo within 24 hours of admission. The initiation of empagliflozin was noted to improve diuresis with increased urinary output and had a significant decrease in the combined endpoint of in-hospital worsening HF, death, and hospital readmission within 60 days. The exact mechanism of benefit of this class remains debated but is thought to be related to the natriuresis promotion without associated RAAS activation and sympathetic tone. It is important to note that nondiabetic patients are not at an increased risk for hypoglycemic events. SGLT2i exert minimal to no effect on blood pressure but often with the initiation of this class providers must monitor volume status and consider a reduction in patients' diuretic doses.[19] The addition of this class is crucial, as SGLT2i have been found to enable tolerability when prescribed alongside other pillars of GDMT, decreasing risk of hyperkalemia and acute kidney injury (AKI).[19] SGLT2i do not increase patients' risk for urinary tract infections; however, genital mycotic infections have occurred more commonly with this class than placebo.[20]

GUIDELINE-DIRECTED MEDICAL THERAPY SEQUENCING IN SPECIAL POPULATIONS
Rationale for Flexible Sequencing

The conventional approach for GDMT initiation involves increasing each agent to target dosing before the initiation of another agent, and doing so in the "order of discovery": RAASi - > BB - > MRA - > SGLT2i. However, the conventional approach assumes that the effectiveness and tolerability of the GDMT agents (**Table 2**) mirror the order in which they were historically developed, which is not true. In addition, the conventional approach neglects to recognize that the beneficial effect of each drug is additive and independent of prerequisite achievement of target doses of prior drugs. A rigid adherence to this approach will deprive or delay the achievement of full GDMT in certain patients. For instance, McMurray and Packer make a convincing case for the simultaneous initiation of SGLT2i and BB, as SGLT2i are very well-tolerated and do not require dose titration.[21] In the sections that follow, we describe strategies for flexible GDMT sequencing in special patient populations. These clinical phenotypes can be dynamic—patients may transition between different phenotypes over the course of their illness.

The initiation of all four pillars of GDMT takes priority over the optimization of an individual medication to target dosing.[22] GDMT initiated during an inpatient encounter are much more likely to "stick" as chronic outpatient medications. Deferring initiation of GDMT to the outpatient setting is associated with a greater than 75% chance that GDMT will not be started within the next year.[23]

Heart Failure with Reduced Ejection Fraction with Hypotension

It should be noted that low BP may be a reflection of progression of pump failure, overdiuresis, dehydration, ischemia, gastrointestinal bleeding, autonomic dysfunction, infection, or another unrelated pathologic process. In HFrEF patients who have persistent borderline hypotension after the treatment of reversible causes of acute hypotension, SGLT2i and MRA can be first considered, as these medications usually minimally affect blood pressure.

SGLT2i are "smart" diuretics that reduce plasma volume without the compensatory neurohumoral and renin–angiotensin-aldosterone system activation.[24] In DAPA-HF, the rate of discontinuation of dapagliflozin and placebo in patients with baseline SBP of less than 110 mm Hg was no different from that in patients with baseline SBP 110 to 120, SBP 120 to 130, and SBP $\geq$130.[25] In patients with baseline SBP less than 110 mm Hg, the between-treatment difference of dapagliflozin compared with placebo was −1.50 mm Hg at 2 weeks, −1.05 mm Hg at 2 months, and −0.68 mm Hg at 8 months.[25] In EMPULSE, the adjusted mean SBP change was +0.1 mm Hg in

the empagliflozin group and +1.0 mm Hg in the placebo group at 3 months.[17,25,26]

Regarding MRA, pooled data from RALES and EMPHASIS-HF fascinatingly demonstrated an increase in SBP in those with low baseline SBP. At 1 month, patients with baseline SBP $\leq$ 105 mm Hg increased by 6.1 mm Hg in the MRA arm and 8.9 mm Hg in the placebo arm, with a between-treatment difference of 2.8 mm Hg. At 6 months, SBP further increased to 9.6 mm Hg in the MRA arm and 12.3 mm Hg in the placebo arm, with a between-treatment difference of 2.8 mm Hg.[26] Meanwhile, for patients with baseline SBP greater than 135 mm Hg, SBP decreased by 11.9 mm Hg in the MRA arm and decreased by 10.0 mm Hg in the placebo arm, for a mean treatment difference of 1.8 mm Hg; at 6 months, SBP decreased by 13.0 mm Hg in the MRA arm and decreased by 9.3 mm Hg in the placebo arm, for a mean treatment difference of 3.6 mm Hg.[26] Moreover, ATHENA-HF showed no significant difference in the BP or HR change with higher spironolactone dosing than targeted for HFrEF compared with placebo.[27]

RAASi has a greater effect on BP than SGLT2i and MRA. If patients are hypotensive, this drug class can be started at a later time as hemodynamics allow. A distinction should be made between hypotension and low blood pressure due to high SVR. In situations with high SVR, RAASi may be beneficial for afterload reduction despite a low BP. Of note, despite anecdotal experience possibly suggesting the contrary, the blood pressure effect of sacubitril–valsartan is not more potent than that of an ACEI or an ARB. PIONEER-HF showed that in patients with low versus high SBP, there was no difference in symptomatic hypotension with the inpatient initiation of sacubitril/valsartan compared with enalapril.[28]

With regard to choice of BB, historically, carvedilol has been considered to have greater immediate suppressive effect on blood pressure than metoprolol or bisoprolol due to its additional component of alpha-adrenergic receptor antagonism.[29,30] In one trial, carvedilol depressed BP to a greater degree than metoprolol.[31] In COPERNICUS, among patients with a baseline SBP of 85 to 95 mm Hg, the use of carvedilol (from 3.125 mg BID up-titrated as tolerated to 25 mg BID) did not depress BP compared with placebo.[32] In patients who have HR greater than 70 but who cannot tolerate BB, ivabradine can be considered, as ivabradine reduces HR without depressing BP.[5]

In all patients in whom low blood pressure is a challenge to GDMT use, a review should be undertaken to see if alpha blockers, calcium channel blockers, nitrates, PDE-5 inhibitors can be downtitrated or switched to alternative medications for

Table 2
Overview of guideline-directed medical therapy agents by class, target doses, adverse effects, and number needed to treat for improving all-cause mortality

GDMT Class	Study (Year)	Study Design	Size	Key Outcome
RAASi	CONSENSUS (1987)	Randomized patients with severe HFrEF and New York Heart Association (NYHA) class IV symptoms to enalapril vs standard of care	253	Enalapril improved survival in NYHA class IV HFrEF when added to standard therapy.
	PIONEER-HF (2018)	Randomized patients hospitalized with acute decompensated HFrEF to initiation of sacubitril–valsartan vs enalapril	881	Sacubitril–valsartan reduced NT-proBNP compared with enalapril at 4 and 8 wk without significantly different rates of medication-related adverse effects
	LIFE (2021)	Randomized patients with advanced HFrEF (NYHA class IV) to sacubitril/valsartan vs valsartan	335	There was no significant difference between sacubitril/valsartan vs valsartan in reducing NT-proBNP. There was an increase in non-life-threatening hyperkalemia in the sacubitril/valsartan arm. Otherwise, there were no significant observed safety concerns.
BB	COPERNICUS (2002)	Randomized patients with HFrEF <25% and NYHA class III–IV symptoms to carvedilol vs placebo	2289	Carvedilol reduces the risk of death or HF hospitalization by 31% compared with placebo
	IMPACT HF (2004)	Randomized stabilized patients hospitalized for heart failure to carvedilol initiation pre-discharge vs post-discharge initiation (> 2 weeks)	363	Initiation of BB with carvedilol pre-discharge was associated with increased beta blocker use at 60-d follow-up, compared with initiation of BB therapy after discharge at the discretion of the physician
MRA	EPHESUS (2003)	Randomized patients with acute myocardial infarction (MI) complicated by left ventricle (LV) dysfunction and HF symptoms to eplerenone vs placebo	6642	Eplerenone reduced mortality among patients with acute MI complicated by LV dysfunction and HF symptoms
SGLT-2	SOLOIST-WHF (2021)	Randomized patients with type II diabetes mellitus (DM-2) who were recently hospitalized for worsening heart failure to sotagliflozin vs placebo	1222	Sotagliflozin, initiated before or shortly after discharge, was associated with significantly lower cardiovascular mortality and HF hospitalizations or urgent care visits for HF compared with placebo
	EMPULSE (2022)	Randomized patients with acute decompensated HF (regardless of left ventricular ejection fraction [LVEF]) to empagliflozin vs placebo	530	Initiation of empagliflozin was associated with significant clinical benefit at 90 d in patients hospitalized for acute HF. Clinical benefits are defined as a hierarchical composite of death from any cause, number of HF events, and time to first HF event, or ≥ 5 points difference in change from baseline in the Kansas City Cardiomyopathy Questionnaire (KCCQ)
ACEi/ARB/ ARNi; BB and MRA	STONG-HF (2022)	Randomized admitted patients with acute HF who are not on full doses of GDMT to high-intensity up-titration vs usual care	1078	Rapid up-titration of GDMT with close follow-up was safe and associated with reduced risk of 180-d all-cause mortality or HF readmission compared with the usual care

their respective indications. Blood pressure-affecting medications can be retimed and staggered from each other. It is important to treat the patient, not the blood pressure, as it is possible for HFrEF patients to tolerate GDMT despite low BP measurements. It is not uncommon for BP to transiently decrease, especially in the first 2 to 4 hours after administration of a GDMT agent, but medium- and long-term BP changes seem to remain stable. If a patient is free of hypotensive symptoms, such as lightheadedness, GDMT can be continued even if SBP is between 80 and 100 mm Hg.[33]

Heart Failure with Reduced Ejection Fraction with Chronic Kidney Disease

Patients with chronic kidney disease (CKD) are prone to hemodynamic AKI and hyperkalemia, which are common barriers to GDMT initiation/up-titration, but they also represent the subgroup that reaps the most benefit from GDMT.[34] Randomized control trials largely excluded patients with HFrEF advanced CKD, but evidence from recent years have offered reassurance. SGLT2i are renoprotective agents that should be initiated early if the eGFR is $\geq$ 20 mL/min/1.73 m^2. DAPA-CKD[35] and SCORED[36] had enrolled CKD patients with eGFR $\geq$25 mL/min/1.73 m^2, whereas EMPA-KIDNEY, EMPEROR-Reduced,[37] and EMPEROR-Preserved[38] enrolled participants with eGFR $\geq$20 mL/min/1.73 m^2. In DAPA-CKD, dapagliflozin was continued even when eGFR declined to less than 15 mL/min per 1.73 m^2.[39] The Kidney Disease Improving Global Outcomes (KDIGO) 2022 guidelines advocate for the use of SGLT2i even if eGFR reaches less than 20 mL/min/1.73 m^2, until renal replacement therapy is started.[40]

BBs can be initiated and continued during CKD at any time. Observational study from the Swedish Heart Failure Registry showed that BB improved survival in this patient population. Further, BB use decreases cardiovascular mortality and HF hospitalization in CKD patients, with a better outcome in patients with eGFR less than 15 mL/min/1.73 m^2 than in those with an eGFR between 15 and less than 30 mL/min/1.73 m^2.[41]

RAASi should be started if the patients' eGFR is greater than 30 mL/min/1.73 m^2 and potassium is less than 5.0 mmol/L.[42] Specialist supervision and laboratory monitoring in a week after RAASi initiation are warranted in patients with stage 4 or higher CKD. RAASi should not be routinely discontinued even if the eGFR falls below 30 mL/min/1.73 m^2 given the survival benefit with the use of RAASi in CKD patients.[43]

In contrast to the other GDMT agents, MRA is less flexible in CKD. MRA is permitted for eGFR of $\geq$30 mL/min/1.73 m^2 as long as potassium is $\leq$ 5.0 mEq/L, which means that most patients with CKD 4, 5, and end stage kidney disease (ESKD) will not be expected to be on an MRA. Finerenone, non-steroidal MRA has been shown to confer renoprotection in patients with diabetic kidney disease; however, non-steroidal MRA have not been shown to be able to effectively replace steroidal MRA (eg, spironolactone) for the treatment of HFrEF.[40]

Heart Failure with Reduced Ejection Fraction with Worsening Renal Function

WRF after initiation of GDMT should be evaluated in the context of the overall clinical picture. Clinical reasoning is of paramount importance to avoid reflexive discontinuation of GDMT in the name of "acute kidney injury" and the labeling of RAASi as "nephrotoxins."[44] Increasing serum creatinine for patients with HFrEF in the setting of aggressive diuresis and initiation of SGLT2i or RAASi has not only been shown to normalize with time but also confers favorable outcomes in the long term.[45,46] In an analysis of HFrEF patients who received enalapril in SOLVD, enalapril-associated eGFR decline of up to 35% has been associated with reduced HF hospitalization rates; enalapril-associated eGFR decline of up to 15% has been associated improved mortality.[45] Given the protective effect of RAASi for cardiovascular events and mortality, discontinuation of RAASi should be temporary, and to be resumed before discharge.

In EMPA-REG OUTCOME, one-third of the HFrEF patients who were given empagliflozin experienced a decrease in eGFR by greater than 10% within the first 4 weeks. However, eGFR eventually stabilized at week 4, including in patients who had an initial drop in eGFR exceeding 30%.[46] In contrast, patients who were given placebo continued to have a decline in their GFR.[46] Moreover, patients with an eGFR dip did not experience an impact on the treatment effect of empagliflozin on subsequent cardiovascular mortality, HF hospitalization, or incident/worsening kidney disease.

The key is to distinguish between transient WRF on initiation of SGLT2i/RAASi versus AKI or acute tubular injury (ATI). In patients with AKI/ATI, optimization of volume status is imperative to avoid mortality associated with fluid overload. BB can be continued throughout AKI. The same cannot be said for MRA. Given the risk of hyperkalemia with declining renal function, MRA should be deferred until AKI is resolved.

Heart Failure with Reduced Ejection Fraction with Hyperkalemia

Hyperkalemia is common in patients with HFrEF, CKD, and in those receiving RAASi.[47] In these patients, SGLT2i or BB may be most amenable to initiation compared with MRA or RAASi. SGLT2i may enhance kaliuresis through the delivery of sodium to the distal convoluted tubule, activation of tubuloglomerular feedback, activation of RAAS, and secretion of aldosterone, which excrete potassium.[48] Evidence from CREDENCE showed that in CKD patients taking RAASi, canagliflozin actually reduced the risk of hyperkalemia by 23%.[49] BB could be started concurrently with SGT2i in patients with hyperkalemia, as there is no mechanism for BBs to cause hyperkalemia. Post hoc analysis from CAPRICORN and COPERNICUS showed that in CKD patients taking carvedilol, the risk of hyperkalemia was only 2%.[50]

In contrast, RAASi and MRA should be reserved later in GDMT sequencing among patients with hyperkalemia risk. Current HF guidelines advise against MRA use in patients with serum potassium levels greater than 5.0 mEq/L.[42] In regard to RAASi, RESOLVD showed that compared with ACEI, ARB had significantly lower serum potassium, without a change in creatinine level. ELITE similarly showed that in HFrEF patients, the risk of hyperkalemia is higher in ACEIs than ARBs.[51] There was an increase in Ang II with ARB, but the level of aldosterone was similar to that of ACEi.[52]

Acute hyperkalemia during hospitalization should be managed with conventional treatments which include insulin, beta-agonist, diuretics, and potassium binders. In chronic hyperkalemia, the management strategies vary according to region and provider preference. Potassium binders include sodium polystyrene sulfonate, sodium zirconium cyclosilicate (SZC), and patiromer. For patients with and without CKD, SZC significantly reduced potassium levels more than placebo.[53] As SZC works as a sodium/potassium exchanger in the gut, there is concern for volume overload.[54] However, adverse volume effects of SZC including hypertension, weight gain, and edema during hyperkalemia treatment have not been observed. OPAL-HK, which enrolled patients with stages 3 or 4 CKD and serum potassium of 5.1 to 6.5 mEq/L, showed that patiromer was associated with a significant reduction in serum potassium levels (-1.01 ± 0.03 mEq/L) and less recurrence of hyperkalemia.[55] PEARL-HF enrolled 107 HF patients and found that over 90% of the patients receiving patiromer were able to reach the target dose of spironolactone.[56] In DIAMOND, which studied HFrEF patients with eGFR $\geq$30 mL/min/ 1.73 m^2, compared with placebo, the patiromer treatment group experienced lower incident hyperkalemia and was more likely to continue MRAs than the placebo group; 95% of patients in the treatment group achieved target dose MRA.[57] The number-needed-to-treat (NNT) with patiromer for HFrEF patients with a history of hyperkalemia to avoid one MRA preventable cardiovascular death or hospitalization over 3 years is more than 400.[58] Future studies would need to evaluate the cost-effective and long-term safety of potassium binders in chronic hyperkalemia.

The concept of prioritizing GDMT enabling therapies recognizes that certain medications allow for a higher permissibility or tolerance of side effects from subsequent GDMT classes.[19] For example, post hoc analysis of the PARADIGM-HF (**Fig. 1**) trial showed that compared with enalapril, sacubitril–valsartan was associated with a reduced risk of hyperkalemia in patients receiving MRAs and fewer discontinuations of MRAs.[59] Data from EMPEROR-Pooled (both the EMPEROR-Reduced and EMPEROR-Preserved combined) showed that empagliflozin reduced hyperkalaemia and new initiation of potassium binders; the effect is greater among patients with lower eGFR and among those with a recent HF hospitalization.[60]

Heart Failure with Reduced Ejection Fraction with Atrial Fibrillation

The management of patients with HFrEF and atrial fibrillation (AF) should prioritize optimization of GDMT over the decision of choosing rate versus rhythm control.[61] With regard to choice of AV nodal blockade, BB is preferred over non-dihydropyridine calcium channel blocker (DHP CCB), because CCB is not a component of HFrEF GDMT, and non-DHP CCBs are harmful in HFrEF due to their negative inotropic effects.[5] Similarly, sotalol, flecainide, disopyramide, and dronedarone are contraindicated in HFrEF.[5] The control of AF can improve control of HFrEF and vice versa. Hypervolemic patients with AF should undergo aggressive diuresis, as decongestion would counter the sympathetic drive, slow down the ventricular rate, and increase the success of conversion to sinus rhythm.

Although BBs would ideally be the first agent in this setting ahead of RAASi or MRA, lenient rate control is preferred for HFrEF patients with comorbid AF. Although resting heart rate is associated with cardiovascular mortality and HF hospitalization in HFrEF patients in sinus rhythm, the relationship does not hold true in HFrEF patients with AF.[62] Although guidelines recommend that HFrEF patients in sinus rhythm maintain a resting heart rate

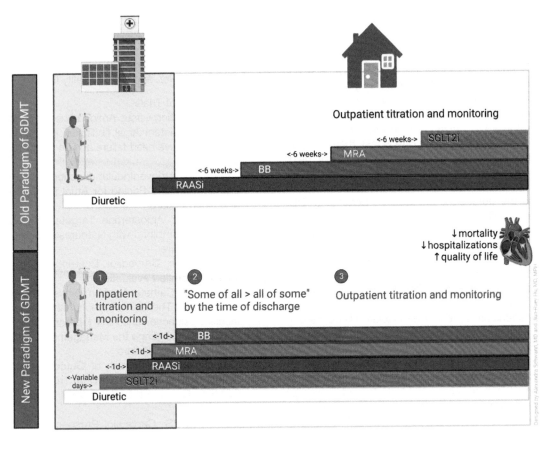

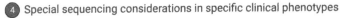

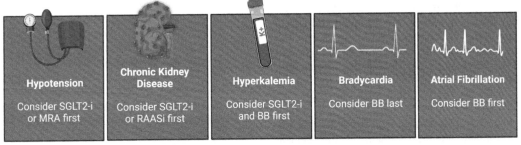

Fig. 1. Figure displaying the contrast of the old vs. new paradigms of GDMT initiation with special sequencing considerations in specific clinical phenotypes. (Created with BioRender.com.)

in the 60s,[5] there is no agreement for the optimal target heart rate for HFrEF patients with AF.[63] The guideline recommendation for using ivabradine to achieve HR less than 70 (Class IIa) only applies to HFrEF patients in sinus rhythm (SR), not HFrEF patients with AF.[5] Patient-level meta-analyses of trials with BB versus placebo in HFrEF found that BB led to a reduction in all-cause mortality and cardiovascular mortality in patients in sinus rhythm, but not in patients with AF.[64,65]

In HFrEF patients with symptomatic AF, ablation is reasonable for improving symptoms and quality of life (Class IIa), as AATAC and CASTLE AF showed a reduction in hospitalization and mortality in HFrEF patients who underwent AF ablation.[66,67] The APAF-CRT mortality trial showed that AV junction ablation plus biventricular pacemaker placement improved survival compared with strict pharmacologic rate control in both patients with HFrEF and patients with HFpEF AV nodal ablation and CRT implantation.[68] Ablation may also pave the way for greater flexibility in deploying HFrEF medications.

Heart Failure with Reduced Ejection Fraction with Bradycardia

For management of HF patients with bradycardia, BB should be sequenced after RAASi, SGLT2i, and MRA, none of which significantly impact heart rate. A medication review should include the consideration of de-prescribing nonessential drugs that have a negative chronotropic effect, such as non-DHP CCBs. If heart rate is less than 50 bpm, BB and ivabradine should be reduced or held. Pacemaker implantation can be considered to allow for up-titration of GDMT,[5] and so as not to lose the adrenergic antagonism benefits of BB. The GDMT class whose mortality benefit is most dose-dependent is BB, although there is value in up-titrating all classes of GDMT, the most value arises from up-titrating BB.[69] With regard to choice of BB, bisoprolol has the greatest immediate suppressive effect on heart rate, followed by metoprolol, then carvedilol,[29,30,70,71] suggesting that if hypertension is present with isolated bradycardia, carvedilol can be considered the evidence-based BB of choice. However, in the long term, there may be no difference in heart rate lowering among individual BB selections. In COMET, a randomized comparison of metoprolol tartrate and carvedilol found a miniscule difference in heart rate at 4 months (<2 bpm) with no difference at 16 months.

SUMMARY

GDMT works. Does the sequence in which GDMT matter? Yes—if it increases the permissibility of initiating the remaining GDMT agents; No—in most other cases, as long as all recommended classes of therapy are eventually prescribed. What matters most is that all patients with HFrEF should be treated with four pillars of GDMT as soon as possible; furthermore, clinicians should endeavor to rapidly titrate these therapies to target or maximally tolerated dosing at the earliest possible occasion. Along with an overview of the safety, efficacy, and tolerability of GDMT, we have carefully discussed several clinical scenarios in which the sequence of GDMT implementation is especially relevant. At times, insightful clinical acumen is necessary for the successful initiation and titration of these medication classes to ensure optimal outcomes for patients with HFrEF. The acute care setting affords a unique, closely monitored environment with emerging evidence to support the safety and effectiveness of intensive GDMT management in stabilized AHF patients. As long as GDMT is initiated appropriately, it is quite safe and well tolerated—even among patients hospitalized with HFrEF. Developing strategies to overcome therapeutic inertia and to achieve maximally tolerated doses of GDMT should be a common goal of all clinicians caring for patients with HFrEF, as GDMT enables patients with HFrEF to live longer, healthier, and higher quality lives.

Abbreviations of Trials
- AATAC: Ablation versus Amiodarone for Treatment of persistent Atrial fibrillation in patients with Congestive heart failure and an implanted device
- APAF-CRT: Atrioventricular Junction Ablation and Biventricular Pacing for Atrial Fibrillation and Heart Failure
- ATHENA-HF: Aldosterone Targeted Neurohormonal Combined with Natriuresis Therapy in Heart Failure
- CAPRICORN: CArvedilol Post-infaRct surVIval COntRolled evaluatioN
- CASTLE-AF: Catheter Ablation versus Standard Conventional Therapy in Patients with Left Ventricular Dysfunction and Atrial Fibrillation
- CHAMP-HF: Change the Management of Patients with Heart Failure
- COACH-HF: Comparison of Outcomes and Access to Care for Heart Failure Trial
- COMET: Carvedilol Or Metoprolol European Trial
- COPERNICUS: Carvedilol Prospective Randomized Cumulative Survival
- CREDENCE: Canagliflozin and Renal Events in Diabetes with Established Nephropathy Clinical Evaluation
- DAPA-CKD: Dapagliflozin and Prevention of Adverse Outcomes in Chronic Kidney Disease
- DAPA-HF: Dapagliflozin and Prevention of Adverse Outcomes in Heart Failure
- DIAMOND: Patiromer for the Management of Hyperkalemia in Subjects Receiving RAASi Medications for the Treatment of Heart Failure
- EMPA-KIDNEY: The Study of Heart and Kidney Protection With Empagliflozin
- EMPA-REG OUTCOME: Empagliflozin Cardiovascular Outcome Event Trial in Type 2 Diabetes Mellitus Patients
- EMPA-RESPONSE-AHF: Randomized, Double-Blind, Placebo-Controlled, Multicenter Pilot Study on the Effects of Empagliflozin on Clinical Outcomes in Patients With Acute Decompensated Heart Failure
- EMPEROR-Reduced: EMPagliflozin outcomE tRial in Patients With chrOnic heaRt Failure With Reduced Ejection Fraction
- EMPEROR-Preserved: Empagliflozin Outcome Trial in Patients with Chronic Heart Failure with Preserved Ejection Fraction

- EMPHASIS-HF: Eplerenone in Mild Patients Hospitalization and Survival Study in Heart Failure
- EMPULSE: EMPagliflozin 10 mg Compared to Placebo, Initiated in Patients Hospitalised for acUte Heart faiLure (de Novo or Decompensated Chronic HF) Who Have Been StabilisEd
- ELITE: Evaluation of Losartan in the Elderly Study
- IMPACT-HF: Initiation Management Predischarge Process for Assessment of Carvedilol Therapy for Heart Failure
- OPAL-HK: A Two-Part, Single-Blind, Phase 3 Study Evaluating the Efficacy and Safety of Patiromer for the Treatment of Hyperkalemia
- PARADIGM-HF: Prospective comparison of ARNI with ACEI to Determine Impact on Global Mortality and morbidity in Heart Failure
- PEARL-HF: Multicenter, Randomized, Double-blind, Placebo-Controlled, Parallel-Group, Multiple-Dose to Evaluate the Effects of RLY5016 in Heart Failure Patients
- PIONEER-HF: Comparison of Sacubitril/Valsartan Versus Enalapril on Effect on NT-proBNP in Patients Stabilized From an Acute Heart Failure Episode
- Potassium Reduction Initiative to Optimize RAAS Inhibition Therapy With Sodium Zirconium Cyclosilicate in Heart Failure
- RALES: Randomized Aldactone Evaluation Study
- SCORED: Effect of Sotagliflozin on Cardiovascular and Renal Events in Patients with Type 2 Diabetes and Moderate Renal Impairment Who Are at Cardiovascular Risk
- SOLVD: Studies of Left Ventricular Dysfunction
- STRONG-HF: Safety, tolerability and efficacy of up-titration of guideline-directed medical therapies for acute heart failure

CLINICS CARE POINTS

- Guideline directed medical therapy is a life saving intervention for patients with heart failure with reduced ejection fraction. It is imperative that patients with this disease be provided with these disease modifying therapies.
- The order by which forms of guideline directed medical therapy are initiated matters less than the end result whereby patients with heart failure with reduced ejection fraction have been started on all four pillars of therapy.
- Special sequencing considerations in specific clinical phenotypes can allow for the ultimate goal of achieving initiation of all four pillars

of guideline directed medical therapy in patients with heart failure with reduced ejection fraction.

DISCLOSURE

No grants, contracts, or other forms of financial support were received for this article. Dr Ralph Riello is on the advisory board of AstraZeneca, Janssen and Johnson & Johnson and has received honoraria/consultation fees from Janssen, Johnson & Johnson, and Pfizer. All remaining authors have no disclosures.

REFERENCES

1. Halliday BP, Wassall R, Lota AS, et al. Withdrawal of pharmacological treatment for heart failure in patients with recovered dilated cardiomyopathy (TRED-HF): an open-label, pilot, randomised trial. Lancet 2019; 393(10166):61–73.
2. Heidenreich PA, Bozkurt B, Aguilar D, et al. 2022 AHA/ACC/HFSA guideline for the management of heart failure: a report of the American College of Cardiology/American heart association joint Committee on clinical practice guidelines. J Am Coll Cardiol 2022;79(17):e263–421.
3. Tan J, Hu JR. GDMT for Everyone. Guideline-Directed Medical Therapy for Everyone. Published May 2022. Available at: www.GDMT.org. Accessed January 31, 2023.
4. Mebazaa A, Davison B, Chioncel O, et al. Safety, tolerability and efficacy of up-titration of guideline-directed medical therapies for acute heart failure (STRONG-HF): a multinational, open-label, randomised, trial. Lancet 2022. https://doi.org/10.1016/S0140-6736(22)02076-1.
5. Heidenreich PA, Bozkurt B, Aguilar D, et al. 2022 AHA/ACC/HFSA guideline for the management of heart failure: a report of the American College of Cardiology/American heart association joint Committee on clinical practice guidelines. Circulation 2022;145(18):e895–1032.
6. Velazquez EJ, Morrow DA, DeVore AD, et al. Angiotensin–neprilysin inhibition in acute decompensated heart failure. N Engl J Med 2019;380(6):539–48.
7. Gattis WA, O'Connor CM, Gallup DS, et al. IMPACT-HF Investigators and Coordinators. Predischarge initiation of carvedilol in patients hospitalized for decompensated heart failure: results of the initiation management Predischarge: process for assessment of carvedilol therapy in heart failure (IMPACT-HF) trial. J Am Coll Cardiol 2004;43(9):1534–41.
8. Ko DT, Hebert PR, Coffey CS, et al. Adverse effects of β-blocker therapy for patients with heart failure: a

quantitative overview of randomized trials. Arch Intern Med 2004;164(13):1389–94.

9. Greene SJ, Butler J, Albert NM, et al. Medical therapy for heart failure with reduced ejection fraction: the CHAMP-HF Registry. J Am Coll Cardiol 2018; 72(4):351–66.

10. Eschalier R, McMurray JJV, Swedberg K, et al. Safety and efficacy of Eplerenone in patients at high risk for hyperkalemia and/or worsening renal function: analyses of the EMPHASIS-HF study subgroups (Eplerenone in Mild patients hospitalization and SurvIval study in heart failure). J Am Coll Cardiol 2013;62(17):1585–93.

11. Maisel A, Xue Y, van Veldhuisen DJ, et al. Effect of spironolactone on 30-day death and heart failure rehospitalization (from the COACH study). Am J Cardiol 2014;114(5):737–42.

12. Butler J, Anstrom KJ, Felker GM, et al. Efficacy and safety of spironolactone in acute heart failure: the ATHENA-HF randomized clinical trial. JAMA Cardiol 2017;2(9):950–8.

13. Butler J, Anker SD, Lund LH, et al. Patiromer for the management of hyperkalemia in heart failure with reduced ejection fraction: the DIAMOND trial. Eur Heart J 2022;43(41):4362–73.

14. Buysse JM, Huang IZ, Pitt B. PEARL-HF: prevention of hyperkalemia in patients with heart failure using a novel polymeric potassium binder, RLY5016. Future Cardiol 2012;8(1):17–28.

15. Vukadinović D, Lavall D, Vukadinović AN, et al. True rate of mineralocorticoid receptor antagonists-related hyperkalemia in placebo-controlled trials: a meta-analysis. Am Heart J 2017;188:99–108.

16. Struthers A, Krum H, Williams GH. A comparison of the aldosterone-blocking agents Eplerenone and spironolactone. Clin Cardiol 2008;31(4):153–8.

17. Voors AA, Angermann CE, Teerlink JR, et al. The SGLT2 inhibitor empagliflozin in patients hospitalized for acute heart failure: a multinational randomized trial. Nat Med 2022;28(3):568–74.

18. Zannad F, Ferreira JP, Pocock SJ, et al. SGLT2 inhibitors in patients with heart failure with reduced ejection fraction: a meta-analysis of the EMPEROR-Reduced and DAPA-HF trials. Lancet Lond Engl 2020;396(10254):819–29.

19. Greene SJ, Butler J, Metra M. Another reason to embrace quadruple medical therapy for heart failure: medications enabling tolerance of each other. Eur J Heart Fail 2021;23(9):1525–8.

20. Lega IC, Bronskill SE, Campitelli MA, et al. Sodium glucose cotransporter 2 inhibitors and risk of genital mycotic and urinary tract infection: a population-based study of older women and men with diabetes. Diabetes Obes Metab 2019;21(11):2394–404.

21. McMurray JJV, Packer M. How should we sequence the treatments for heart failure and a reduced ejection fraction? Circulation 2021;143(9):875–7.

22. Bozkurt B. How to initiate and uptitrate GDMT in heart failure: practical stepwise approach to optimization of GDMT. JACC Heart Fail 2022;10(12): 992–5.

23. Greene SJ, Butler J, Fonarow GC. Simultaneous or rapid sequence initiation of quadruple medical therapy for heart failure—optimizing therapy with the need for speed. JAMA Cardiol 2021;6(7):743–4.

24. Griffin M, Rao VS, Ivey-Miranda J, et al. Empagliflozin in heart failure. Circulation 2020;142(11):1028–39.

25. Serenelli M, Böhm M, Inzucchi SE, et al. Effect of dapagliflozin according to baseline systolic blood pressure in the Dapagliflozin and Prevention of Adverse Outcomes in Heart Failure trial (DAPA-HF). Eur Heart J 2020;41(36):3402–18.

26. Serenelli M, Jackson A, Dewan P, et al. Mineralocorticoid receptor antagonists, blood pressure, and outcomes in heart failure with reduced ejection fraction. Jacc Heart Fail 2020;8(3):188–98.

27. Butler J, Anstrom KJ, Felker GM, et al. Efficacy and safety of spironolactone in acute heart failure. JAMA Cardiol 2017;2(9):950–8.

28. Berg DD, Samsky MD, Velazquez EJ, et al. Efficacy and safety of sacubitril/valsartan in high-risk patients in the PIONEER-HF trial. Circ Heart Fail 2021;14(2): e007034.

29. Stoschitzky K, Stoschitzky G, Brussee H, et al. Comparing beta-blocking effects of bisoprolol, carvedilol and nebivolol. Cardiology 2006;106(4): 199–206.

30. Stoschitzky K, Koshucharova G, Zweiker R, et al. Differing beta-blocking effects of carvedilol and metoprolol. Eur J Heart Fail 2001;3(3):343–9.

31. Sanderson JE, Chan SK, Yip G, et al. Beta-blockade in heart failure: a comparison of carvedilol with metoprolol. J Am Coll Cardiol 1999;34(5):1522–8.

32. Rouleau JL, Roecker EB, Tendera M, et al. Influence of pretreatment systolic blood pressure on the effect of carvedilol in patients with severe chronic heart failure: the Carvedilol Prospective Randomized Cumulative Survival (COPERNICUS) study. J Am Coll Cardiol 2004;43(8):1423–9.

33. Bozkurt B. Response to Ryan and Parwani: heart failure patients with low blood pressure: How should we manage neurohormonal blocking drugs? Circ Heart Fail 2012;5(6):820–1.

34. Vaduganathan M, Fonarow GC, Greene SJ, et al. Treatment persistence of renin-angiotensin-aldosterone-system inhibitors over time in heart failure with reduced ejection fraction. J Card Fail 2022; 28(2):191–201.

35. Heerspink HJL, Stefánsson BV, Correa-Rotter R, et al. Dapagliflozin in patients with chronic kidney disease. N Engl J Med 2020;383(15):1436–46.

36. Bhatt DL, Szarek M, Steg PG, et al. Sotagliflozin in patients with diabetes and recent worsening heart failure. N Engl J Med 2021;384(2):117–28.

37. Packer M, Anker SD, Butler J, et al. Cardiovascular and renal outcomes with empagliflozin in heart failure. N Engl J Med 2020;383(15):1413–24.

38. Anker SD, Butler J, Filippatos G, et al. Empagliflozin in heart failure with a preserved ejection fraction. N Engl J Med 2021;385(16):1451–61.

39. Chertow GM, Vart P, Jongs N, et al. Effects of dapagliflozin in stage 4 chronic kidney disease. J Am Soc Nephrol 2021;32(9):2352–61.

40. Rossing P, Caramori ML, Chan JCN, et al. Executive summary of the KDIGO 2022 clinical practice guideline for diabetes management in chronic kidney disease: an update based on rapidly emerging new evidence. Kidney Int 2022;102(5):990–9.

41. Fu EL, Uijl A, Dekker FW, et al. Association between β-blocker use and mortality/morbidity in patients with heart failure with reduced, midrange, and preserved ejection fraction and advanced chronic kidney disease. Circ Heart Fail 2020;13(11):e007180.

42. Yancy CW, Jessup M, Bozkurt B, et al. 2017 ACC/AHA/HFSA focused update of the 2013 ACCF/AHA guideline for the management of heart failure: a report of the American College of Cardiology/American heart association task force on clinical practice guidelines and the heart failure society of America. J Card Fail 2017;23(8):628–51.

43. Kidney Disease: Improving Global Outcomes (KDIGO) CKD Work Group. KDIGO 2012 clinical practice guideline for the evaluation and management of chronic kidney disease. Kidney Int 2013; Suppl(3):1–150.

44. Bozkurt B. The need to stop Inappropriate Coding for acute kidney injury in heart failure. JACC Heart Fail 2022;10(9):692–4.

45. McCallum W, Tighiouart H, Ku E, et al. Acute declines in estimated glomerular filtration rate on enalapril and mortality and cardiovascular outcomes in patients with heart failure with reduced ejection fraction. Kidney Int 2019;96(5):1185–94.

46. Kraus BJ, Weir MR, Bakris GL, et al. Characterization and implications of the initial estimated glomerular filtration rate 'dip' upon sodium-glucose cotransporter-2 inhibition with empagliflozin in the EMPA-REG OUTCOME trial. Kidney Int 2021;99(3):750–62.

47. Jain N, Kotla S, Little BB, et al. Predictors of hyperkalemia and death in patients with cardiac and renal disease. Am J Cardiol 2012;109(10):1510–3.

48. Heerspink HJL, Perkins BA, Fitchett DH, et al. Sodium glucose cotransporter 2 inhibitors in the treatment of diabetes mellitus. Circulation 2016; 134(10):752–72.

49. Neuen BL, Oshima M, Perkovic V, et al. Effects of canagliflozin on serum potassium in people with diabetes and chronic kidney disease: the CREDENCE trial. Eur Heart J 2021;42(48):4891–901.

50. Wali RK, Iyengar M, Beck GJ, et al. Efficacy and safety of carvedilol in treatment of heart failure with chronic kidney disease. Circ Heart Fail 2011;4(1): 18–26.

51. Pitt B, Segal R, Martinez FA, et al. Randomised trial of losartan versus captopril in patients over 65 with heart failure (Evaluation of Losartan in the Elderly Study, ELITE). Lancet 1997;349(9054):747–52.

52. McKelvie RS, Yusuf S, Pericak D, et al. Comparison of Candesartan, enalapril, and their Combination in Congestive heart failure. Circulation 1999;100(10): 1056–64.

53. Packham DK, Rasmussen HS, Lavin PT, et al. Sodium zirconium cyclosilicate in hyperkalemia. N Engl J Med 2015;372(3):222–31.

54. Lokelma® (sodium zirconium cyclosilicate) [prescribing information]. Wilmington, DE: AstraZeneca Pharmaceuticals LP; 2022.

55. Weir MR, Bakris GL, Bushinsky DA, et al. Patiromer in patients with kidney disease and hyperkalemia receiving RAAS inhibitors. N Engl J Med 2015; 372(3):211–21.

56. Pitt B, Anker SD, Bushinsky DA, et al. Evaluation of the efficacy and safety of RLY5016, a polymeric potassium binder, in a double-blind, placebo-controlled study in patients with chronic heart failure (the PEARL-HF) trial. Eur Heart J 2011;32(7):820–8.

57. Tromp J, Ouwerkerk W, van Veldhuisen DJ, et al. A systematic review and network meta-analysis of pharmacological treatment of heart failure with reduced ejection fraction. JACC Heart Fail 2022; 10(2):73–84.

58. Packer M. Potassium binders for patients with heart failure? The real enlightenment of the DIAMOND trial. Eur Heart J 2022;43(41):4374–7.

59. Desai AS, Vardeny O, Claggett B, et al. Reduced risk of hyperkalemia during treatment of heart failure with mineralocorticoid receptor antagonists by use of sacubitril/valsartan compared with enalapril: a secondary analysis of the PARADIGM-HF trial. JAMA Cardiol 2017;2(1):79–85.

60. Ferreira JP, Zannad F, Butler J, et al. Empagliflozin and serum potassium in heart failure: an analysis from EMPEROR-Pooled. Eur Heart J 2022;43(31): 2984–93.

61. Lee JZ, Cha YM. Atrial fibrillation and heart failure: a contemporary review of current management approaches. Heart Rhythm O2 2021;2(6):762–70. Part B).

62. Docherty KF, Shen L, Castagno D, et al. Relationship between heart rate and outcomes in patients in sinus rhythm or atrial fibrillation with heart failure and reduced ejection fraction. Eur J Heart Fail 2020; 22(3):528–38.

63. Bauersachs J, Veltmann C. Heart rate control in heart failure with reduced ejection fraction: the bright and the dark side of the moon. Eur J Heart Fail 2020;22(3):539–42.

64. Cleland JGF, Bunting KV, Flather MD, et al. Beta-blockers for heart failure with reduced, mid-range,

and preserved ejection fraction: an individual patient-level analysis of double-blind randomized trials. Eur Heart J 2018;39(1):26–35.

65. Kotecha D, Holmes J, Krum H, et al. Efficacy of β blockers in patients with heart failure plus atrial fibrillation: an individual-patient data meta-analysis. Lancet 2014;384(9961):2235–43.

66. Di Biase L, Mohanty P, Mohanty S, et al. Ablation versus Amiodarone for treatment of persistent atrial fibrillation in patients with Congestive heart failure and an implanted device. Circulation 2016;133(17): 1637–44.

67. Marrouche NF, Brachmann J, Andresen D, et al. Catheter ablation for atrial fibrillation with heart failure. N Engl J Med 2018;378(5):417–27.

68. Brignole M, Pentimalli F, Palmisano P, et al. AV junction ablation and cardiac resynchronization for patients with permanent atrial fibrillation and narrow QRS: the APAF-CRT mortality trial. Eur Heart J 2021;42(46):4731–9.

69. Bristow MR, Gilbert EM, Abraham WT, et al. Carvedilol produces dose-related improvements in Left ventricular function and survival in Subjects with chronic heart failure. Circulation 1996;94(11): 2807–16.

70. Stoschitzky K, Donnerer J, Klein W, et al. Different effects of propranolol, bisoprolol, carvedilol and doxazosin on heart rate, blood pressure, and plasma concentrations of epinephrine and norepinephrine. J Clin Basic Cardiol 2003;6(1):69–72.

71. Vittorio TJ, Zolty R, Kasper ME, et al. Differential effects of carvedilol and metoprolol succinate on plasma norepinephrine release and peak exercise heart rate in Subjects with chronic heart failure. J Cardiovasc Pharmacol Ther 2008;13(1):51–7.

Frailty and Its Implications in Heart Failure with Reduced Ejection Fraction
Impact on Prognosis and Treatment

Khawaja M. Talha, MBBS[a], Stephen J. Greene, MD[b],
Javed Butler, MD, MPH, MBA[a,c], Muhammad Shahzeb Khan, MD, MSc[b],*

KEYWORDS

- Frailty • Heart failure • Reduced ejection fraction • Mortality • Guideline-directed medical therapy
- Rehabilitation

KEY POINTS

- Frailty affects approximately 50% of patients with heart failure with reduced ejection fraction (HFrEF).
- The relationship between frailty and HFrEF is bidirectional, with one condition exacerbating the other.
- Contrary to perceived notions, therapies for HFrEF are generally safe and efficacious in frail patients.
- A targeted approach to the implementation of guideline-directed medical therapy in patients with frail HFrEF is required to improve quality of life and increase event-free survival.

Frailty is defined as a diminished overall capacity of an individual to respond appropriately to a stressful event. In heart failure (HF) with reduced ejection fraction (HFrEF), these changes are driven by multiple factors, including age, clinical co-morbidity burden, heightened inflammatory state, symptomatic burden, nutritional deficiencies, and cognitive impairment.[1] Frailty is present in 30% to 60% of the total HFrEF population[2,3] and is associated with 1.5 to 2-fold increased risk of hospitalizations and death.[4] This may be in part due to a lack of optimization of medical therapy and physical rehabilitation in this high-risk cohort due to perceived intolerance, harm, or lack of benefit from guideline-recommended therapeutic approaches. Herein, we discuss the mechanisms underlying frailty in HFrEF, as well as the clinical profile, outcomes, efficacy of therapeutic strategies, and implementation challenges associated with frail patients with HFrEF.

UNDERLYING MECHANISMS OF FRAILTY IN HEART FAILURE

HF is a multi-system syndrome, with the HFrEF subtype characterized by depressed systolic function associated with several cardiovascular and non-cardiovascular co-morbidities that contribute to the development of frailty. HF is also more commonly associated with older age, a subgroup that already has a diminished physical and physiological reserve, and a higher prevalence of sarcopenia and cognitive dysfunction. Moreover, a heightened inflammatory state is

[a] Department of Medicine, University of Mississippi Medical Center, 2500 North State Street, Jackson, MS 39216, USA; [b] Division of Cardiology, Department of Medicine, Duke University Hospital, 2301 Erwin Road, Durham, NC 27710, USA; [c] Baylor Scott & White Research Institute, 3434 Live Oak Street Suite 501, Dallas, TX 75204, USA
* Corresponding author. 2301 Erwin Road, Durham, NC 27710.
E-mail address: shahzeb.khan@duke.edu

Cardiol Clin 41 (2023) 525–536
https://doi.org/10.1016/j.ccl.2023.06.002
0733-8651/23/© 2023 Elsevier Inc. All rights reserved.

present in HF with elevated levels of cytokines, especially in HFrEF.[5] These cytokines exert a deleterious effect on muscle mass leading to sarcopenia and cachexia, with a relative preservation of adiposity.[6] The heightened pro-inflammatory state coupled with multi-organ damage associated with volume overload and hypoxia associated with HF, and the development of other co-morbidities, e.g., chronic kidney disease (CKD), result in loss of physiological reserve which in turn contributes to frailty. Pro-inflammatory markers such as C-reactive protein, tissue necrosis factor, interleukin-1, and interleukin-6, are elevated in HF and elevate the risk of incident HF in older patients[7]; specifically, interleukin-6 has been found to be more prevalent in older patients with a higher burden of cardiovascular co-morbidities and is associated with increased mortality in HF.[8] However, interleukin antagonists such as anakinra were not effective in improving exercise capacity in patients with decompensated HFrEF.[9] Sarcopenia significantly contributes towards frailty and is more prevalent in HF (by ∼20%) compared to the general population, and negatively impacts outcomes. Sarcopenic patients with HF are likely to be older, have higher levels of serum natriuretic peptide levels, and are nutritionally deficient. In a recent report by Konishi and colleagues, lower mean appendicular mass and fat indices (markers of sarcopenia) were associated with an increased risk of adjusted all-cause mortality in patients with HF. Another study also reported a significantly higher rate of mortality in patients with HF with sarcopenia with an elevated risk in patients with HFrEF compared to HF with preserved ejection fraction (HFpEF).[10]

ASSESSMENT OF FRAILTY

Numerous tools have been identified to objectively assess and stratify frailty. A systematic review identified a total of 67 frailty instruments used in clinical research, of which the most used were iterations of the Fried frailty phenotype and the deficit accumulation index.[11] The Fried frailty phenotype[12] comprised of five components, namely shrinking (defined as unintentional weight loss≥ 10 lbs, or >5% of body weight in 1 year), weakness (assess using hand grip strength), poor endurance and energy (assessed using a self-reported scale), slowness (assessed by the time taken to walk 15 feet), and low physical activity (assessed by energy expenditure per week). The phenotypes are stratified as frail (3 or more deficits), prefrail (1 or 2 deficits), or non-frail (no deficits). The score is convenient, does not require comprehensive clinical assessment, and is of great utility to scree

patients at risk for frailty. However, the criteria provide a discrete variable which is unable to assess the severity of prefrailty or frailty, is not reliable for the follow-up assessment of frailty after therapeutic interventions, has limited real-world generalizability, and does not account for cognitive dysfunction. The modified Fried criteria[13] employs a population-independent approach to frailty to improve the generalizability of the scale.

The Clinical Frailty Scale was one of the first approaches for frailty assessment proposed by Rockwood and colleagues.[14] It is a 7-point scale categorizing patient from being in robust health (1) to complete functional dependence on others (7) and incorporates several self-reported and clinically assessed parameters. The scale evolved into a deficit accumulation index model which incorporates at least 30-40 deficits in function, irrespective of the cause or nature of deficit, that an individual accumulates over time with age.[15] Each deficit is required to satisfy 5-point criteria to be eligible for inclusion. The model produces a score, which is a continuous variable, and is stratified into a frailty index, based on severity, that can be serially measured over time to assess changes in frailty status. This instrument requires comprehensive clinical assessment, provides a more real-world measure of frailty and is increasingly used in frailty assessment in HF studies.

CLINICAL PROFILE

Patients with HFrEF and comorbid frailty are a vulnerable, high-risk population that is more likely to be older and have a greater burden of co-morbidities. Women are more likely to be frail in the general population compared with men, which in part is attributed to lower body muscle mass and longer life expectancy. This difference is also prevalent across patients with HF. In a meta-analysis of 29 studies and 8,854 patients with HF,[16] women were found to be at a 26% higher risk of being frail compared with men. These findings are important as women comprise approximately half of all patients with HFrEF and hence form a significant proportion of the prevalent HFrEF burden, further compounded by increased frailty in this subgroup. Patients with baseline cardiovascular co-morbidities with high frailty are also at increased risk of incident HF. Analyses from the PARADIGM-HF (Prospective Comparison of ARNI with ACEI to Determine Impact on Global Mortality and Morbidity in Heart Failure), ATMOSPHERE (Aliskiren Trial of Minimizing Outcomes in Patients With Heart Failure), and FRAGILE-HF (the prevalence and prognostic value of physical and social frailty in geriatric patients hospitalized for HF: a multicenter prospective cohort study) trials reported a higher prevalence of frailty among White patients, with higher blood pressure, heart rate, and body mass index (BMI).[2,17] Both cardiovascular co-morbidities such as CKD, hypertension, diabetes, and non-cardiovascular co-morbidities such as chronic obstructive pulmonary disease were more prevalent in frail patients with HF. Frail patients had higher symptom burden, lower quality of life scores, higher prevalence of NYHA class II and III scores, higher prevalence of depression, and lower literacy. Frail patients are also at a higher risk of incident HF; the LookAHEAD (Action for Health in Diabetes) trial[18] evaluated the association between frailty (assessed using the deficit accumulation approach) and incidence of index HF. Increasing frailty scores, when used as a continuous variable, were associated with higher rates of both incident HFrEF and HFpEF. Sze and colleagues[19] reported that worsening frailty was associated with all-cause mortality and all-cause hospitalizations, which was significant even after adjustment for confounding variables e.g., age, body mass index, hemoglobin, functional class, co-morbidity burden, and renal function.

PROGNOSIS AND OUTCOMES

In a combined analysis of the PARADIGM-HF and ATMOSPHERE trials among 13,265 patients,[2] high frailty indices (as defined by a 42-pont frailty index using a deficit accumulation approach) were found to be associated with an increased risk of the composite of CV death and HF hospitalizations, all-cause deaths, and total HF hospitalizations. Study drug discontinuation was also found to be higher in the frailest population (20%) compared to non-frail patients (14%). However, the drug's treatment effect in the PARADIGM-HF trial was consistent across all frailty subgroups.

The FRAGILE-HF[17] prospectively evaluated the association between baseline characteristics and individual components of frailty assessment with outcomes in non-dependent elderly patients with HF. The study enrolled 416 patients of which 316 (76%) were found to be frail using the Fried criteria, and approximately 50% of patients had LVEF <50%., frail patients had a greater than 2-fold risk of 1-year mortality, and a nearly 2-fold increased risk of 1-year all-cause readmissions. Moreover, a meta-analysis by Yang and colleagues[4] evaluated all-cause mortality (8 studies) and hospitalizations (6 studies) in frail patients compared to non-frail patients with HF. Frailty was found to increase the risk of all-cause mortality (HR 1.54; 95 CI, 1.34–1.75) over a median

follow-up duration of 1.82 years. It also increased the risk of all-cause hospitalizations by a similar magnitude (HR 1.56; 95% CI, 1.36–1.78) over a median follow-up duration of 1.12 years.

A *post hoc* report of the GUIDE-IT (Guiding Evidence-Based Therapy Using Biomarker Intensified Treatment in Heart Failure) trial[20] primarily analyzed the association between frailty (determined by the Rockwood deficit accumulation approach) and clinical outcomes in 879 patients with HFrEF over 12 months. Approximately 56% of patients were categorized as having a high frailty index (FI class 3). Compared to non-frail patients, patients with high frailty were found to have a significantly increased occurrence of the primary composite outcome (43.2% vs 22.7%; HR 1.76 [95% CI,1.20–2.58]) all-cause mortality (20.8% vs 5.5%; HR 2.55 [95% CI, 1.25–5.20]), and HF hospitalization (27.6% vs 21.5%; HR 1.61 [95% CI, 1.08–2.40]). Highly frail patients were less likely to be started on or up-titrated on both triple GDMT (ACEi [angiotensin-converting enzyme inhibitor]/ARB [aniotensin receptor blocker], beta-blocker, and MRA [mineralocorticoid receptor antagonist]) and double GDMT (ACEi/ARB and beta-blocker) compared to non-frail patients. Highly frail patients also had a significantly increased risk of all-cause mortality and HF hospitalizations compared to non-frail patients.

EFFICACY OF HEART FAILURE THERAPIES IN PATIENTS WITH FRAILTY

The presence of frailty is clinically relevant and may make clinicians more reluctant to optimize medical therapy. This hesitation toward therapy may relate largely to concerns over polypharmacy, adverse drug reactions and intolerance, and/or a perception that medical therapy may be less effective in frail patients as compared with non-frail patients. A recent study reported that ambulatory frail patients were less likely to be on triple medical therapy with ACEi/ARB, beta-blocker, and MRA for HFrEF compared to non-frail patients, and were commonly not on target doses of these medications.[19] To date, there has not been a dedicated clinical trial in confirmed frail patients for any drug intervention for HF. Most of the data for the efficacy of these interventions in frail patients have been derived from observational studies and subgroup or *post hoc* analysis of landmark trials. The results of these analyses frequently use age as a surrogate marker of frailty and although limited in some cases by design, they do indicate consistent relative benefits and safety of HF therapies across the spectrum of age and frailty status (**Table 1**).

Table 1
Studies evaluating the efficacy of drug therapy in the management of heart failure

Author, Year	Drug	Study Description	HFrEF Proportion (%)	N	Main Findings
Ahmed,[21] 2007	Digoxin	A *post hoc* analysis of the DIG trial in elderly patients aged ≥ 65 years to evaluate the efficacy of digoxin at high or low serum digoxin levels	87	5548	• Reduction in all-cause mortality, all-cause hospitalizations, and HF hospitalizations in patients with low serum digoxin concentration (0.5–0.9 ng/mL); only reduction in HF hospitalizations with high serum digoxin concentration (>1 ng/mL)
Packer et al,[22] 2001	Beta-blockers	A sub-group analysis of the main randomized trial of carvedilol in severe chronic HFrEF	100	2289	• Similar reduction in the cumulative risk of all-cause death or any hospitalizations in patients aged <65 year and those aged ≥65 years with carvedilol compared to placebo
Erland et al,[24] 2001	Beta-blockers	A *post hoc* analysis of the main CIBIS-II trial in high-risk patients including those aged ≥71 years	100	2647	• Similar reduction in risk of all-cause death and HF hospitalizations in patients aged <71 or ≥71 years with bisoprolol compared to placebo • Significant reduction in risk of pump failure in the ≥71 years group • No reduction in risk of sudden death in the ≥71 years group
Deedwania et al,[23] 2004	Beta-blockers	A *post hoc* analysis of the MERIT-HF trial in HFrEF patients aged ≥65 years	100	1982	• Reduction in all-cause mortality, sudden death, HF hospitalizations, HF-related deaths in patients aged ≥65 and >75 years with metoprolol compared to placebo
Hernandez et al,[25] 2009	Beta-blockers	A retrospective analysis from the OPTIMIZE registry to assess long-term outcomes in patients aged ≥65 years newly initiated on beta-blocker therapy	42	24,689	• Reduction in all-cause hospitalizations and mortality compared to those not treated with beta-blockers

Study	Drug class	Description		Sample size	Key findings
Pitt 1999 [26]	MRA	A sub-group analysis of the main RALES trial stratified by age (< and ≥67 years)	100	1663	• Similar reduction in the risk of all-cause death or any hospitalizations with spironolactone compared to placebo in the <67 and ≥67 years age groups
Pitt 2003 [27]	MRA	A subgroup analysis of the main EPHESUS trial stratified by age (<65 and ≥65 years)	100	6642	• Similar reduction in the risk of all-cause death and cardiovascular deaths with eplerenone compared to placebo in the <65 and ≥65 years age groups
Zannad et al,[28] 2011	MRA	A subgroup analysis of the main EMPHASIS-HF trial stratified by age (<65 and ≥65 years)	100	2737	• Similar reduction in the risk of HF hospitalizations and cardiovascular deaths with eplerenone compared to placebo in the <65 and ≥65 years age groups
Yaku et al,[30] 2019	MRA	A propensity-matched analysis from the Kyoto Heart Failure registry evaluating the use of MRAs in elderly patients (median age 80) recently hospitalized for HF	36	3717	• Reduction in the composite endpoint of HF hospitalizations and mortality in the overall cohort with MRA • Subgroup analysis of patients with EF ≤40% did not have a significant reduction in the primary endpoint
Flather 2000 [31]	ACEi	A patient-level meta-analysis of the SAVE, AIRE, TRACE, SOLVD Treatment, and SOLVD prevention trials for ACEi in HFrEF	100	12,763	• Significant reduction in risk of all-cause death, myocardial infarction, and HF hospitalizations in the 65 to 74 years age group with ACEi compared to placebo; no significant reduction in the >75 years age group
Greene et al,[33] 2021	ARNI	A retrospective analysis from the Get With The Guideline – HF registry evaluating outcomes in hospitalized patients aged ≥65 years with ARNI	100	14,230	• Compared to ACEi/ARB, reduced risk of all-cause mortality with ARNI • Compared to no prescription of ARNI, reduced risk of all-cause mortality and hospitalizations
Butt et al,[34] 2022	SGLT-2 inhibitors	A post hoc analysis of DAPA-HF in elderly patients aged ≥65 years with HFrEF to evaluate the efficacy and safety of dapagliflozin	100	4742	• Reduction in worsening HF and cardiovascular death across all frailty subgroups stratified by frailty index with dapagliflozin compared to placebo

(continued on next page)

Table 1
(*continued*)

Author, Year	Drug	Study Description	HFrEF Proportion (%)	N	Main Findings
Kitzman et al,[38] 2021	Physical rehabilitation	A randomized trial (REHAB-HF) in hospitalized elderly HF patients to assess the efficacy of physical rehabilitation	47	349	• Significant improved in SPPB, quality of life, frailty status, depression, and 6-minute walk test with physical rehabilitation compared to usual care
Pandey et al,[3,18] 2022	Aerobic exercise	A *post hoc* analysis of the HF-ACTION trial in chronic stable HFrEF patients that evaluated the efficacy of aerobic exercise stratified by frailty status	100	2130	• Significant reduction in the primary composite outcome of HF hospitalizations and cardiovascular death with aerobic exercise compared to usual care in frail patients; no significant reduction observed in non-frail patients

Abbreviations: AIRE, acute infarction ramipril efficacy study; ARNI, angiotensin receptor blocker/neprilysin inhibitor; CIBIS II, the cardiac insufficiency bisoprolol study; DAPA-HF, dapagliflozin and prevention of adverse outcomes in heart failure; DIG, digitalis investigation group; EMPHASIS-HF, eplerenone in mild patients hospitalization and survival study in heart failure; EPHESUS, eplerenone in patients with heart failure due to systolic dysfunction complicating acute myocardial infarction; HF-ACTION, a controlled trial investigating outcomes of exercise training; HFrEF, heart failure with reduced ejection fraction; MERIT-HF, Effect of metoprolol CR/XL in chronic heart failure; Metoprolol CR/XL randomised intervention trial in congestive heart failure; MRA, mineralocorticoid receptor antagonists; OPTIMIZE, organized program to initiate lifesaving treatment in hospitalized patients with heart failure; RALES, randomized aldactone evaluation study; REHAB-HF, rehabilitation therapy in older acute heart failure patients; SAVE, survival and ventricular enlargement; SGLT-2, sodium-glucose co-transporter 2; SOLVD, studies of left ventricular dysfunction; TRACE, trandolapril cardiac evaluation.

Digoxin

A *post hoc* analysis of the DIG (Digitalis Investigation Group) trial examined the effects of low (0.5–0.9 ng/mL) and high (≥1 ng/mL) serum digoxin concentration (SDC) in patients aged ≥65 years, compared to those aged <65 years in the management of HF.[21] A total of 5,548 patients (87% aged ≥65 years with LVEF <45%) were analyzed with a median follow-up over ~40 months, digoxin at low SDC in patients aged ≥65 years. Investigators found a significantly reduced risk of all-cause mortality (HR 0.81; 95% CI, 0.68–0.96), all-cause hospitalizations (HR 0.83; 95% CI, 0.73–0.93), and HF hospitalizations (HR 0.71; 95% CI, 0.58–0.86) in elderly patients with low SDC with similar findings reported in the cohort aged <65 years. High SDC was only associated with a significant risk reduction in HF hospitalizations. Findings also suggested that the dose of digoxin was the strongest predictor of SDC in patients aged ≥ 65 years, while diuretic use strongly predicted SDC among patients aged <65 years. Although the main DIG trial was negative for a reduction in mortality outcomes, this analysis indicates that the benefit of digoxin therapy is consistent across both younger and older cohorts, with a higher magnitude of benefit in patients with low SDC.

Beta-Blockers

Subgroup analysis from the landmark randomized trial of carvedilol in patients with HFrEF revealed a similar benefit of drug therapy in patients aged <65 and those aged ≥65 years in reducing the risk of all-cause death and HF hospitalizations.[22] Similarly, *post hoc* analysis from the MERIT-HF (Effect of metoprolol CR/XL in chronic heart failure: Metoprolol CR/XL Randomised Intervention Trial in Congestive Heart Failure) trial that evaluated the use of extended-release metoprolol in HFrEF revealed similar risk reduction in mortality and HF hospitalization endpoints between the <65 and ≥ 65 years age groups, with effect persistent among patients older than 75 years.[23] Another *post hoc* analysis of the CIBIS-II (Cardiac Insufficiency Bisoprolol Study) trial that evaluated the efficacy of bisoprolol in high-risk patients with HFrEF, the drug was found to be efficacious in reducing all-cause mortality and HF hospitalizations in patients aged <71 years and those aged ≥71 years.[24]

In a propensity-matched analysis from the OPTIMIZE-HF (Organized Program to Initiate Life-saving Treatment in Hospitalized Patients with Heart Failure) registry,[25] Hernandez and colleagues evaluated the efficacy of beta-blocker initiation following an HF hospitalization in attenuating mortality and hospitalizations in elderly patients (age >65 years) with HF. The cohort included 3,001 patients with HFrEF who were followed for 1 year following hospitalization to assess changes in all-cause mortality and all-cause hospitalizations between patients who were initiated on beta-blocker (n = 1,800) therapy versus those who were not (n = 1,201). Among the HFrEF cohort with a median age of 78-80, beta-blocker initiation was significantly associated with a reduction in adjusted all-cause mortality (HR 0.77, 95% CI, 0.68–0.87) and all-cause hospitalizations (HR 0.89, 95% CI, 0.80–0.99).

Mineralocorticoid Receptor Antagonists

Sub-group analyses from the RALES (Randomized Aldactone Evaluation Study),[26] EPHESUS (Eplerenone Post-AMI Heart Failure Efficacy and Survival Study),[27] and EMPHASIS-HF (Eplerenone in Mild Patients Hospitalization and Survival Study in Heart Failure)[28] trials did not reveal a significant difference in the treatment effect of mineralocorticoid receptor antagonists (MRA) in patients aged <65 and those aged ≥65 years, although patients aged ≥75 years with post-myocardial infarction HFrEF did not have a significant reduction in all-cause mortality or cardiovascular death/cardiovascular hospitalizations in the EPHESUS trial.[29]

Yaku and colleagues[30] performed a propensity-matched analysis of HF patients from the Kyoto Congestive Heart Failure Registry to evaluate the clinical outcomes associated with MRAs following an HF hospitalization. A total of 3,717 patients with a median age of 80 years regardless of LVEF with acute decompensated HF were included of which 45.1% were prescribed MRA at discharge. The study found a significant reduction in the primary composite endpoint of 1-year all-cause mortality and HF hospitalizations which was majorly attributed to a significant reduction of 1-year cumulative HF hospitalizations, with No reduction in 1-year all-cause mortality. In subgroup analysis, patients with LVEF ≤40% were not found to have a significant association with the primary endpoint, while patients with LVF >40% had a significant reduction in the primary endpoint, with no significant between-group difference.

Renin-Angiotensin Antagonists

A large patient-level meta-analysis of 5 major ACEi trials in HFrEF included analyses of treatment effect stratified by age groups; age group 65 to 74 was found to have a 33% reduction in the composite endpoint of all-cause death, myocardial infarction, and HF hospitalizations with ACEi use; however, a significant reduction was not observed in patients aged 75 years and older.[31] In an observational propensity-matched analysis from the Get With the Guidelines–Heart Failure (GWTG-HF) registry, Gilstrap and colleagues[32] evaluated the association between beta-blockers and renin-angiotensin antagonists use at hospital discharge in patients aged ≥65 years with HFrEF and 30-day and 1-year mortality. This analysis of 48,711 patients found that patients discharged on renin-angiotensin antagonists had a lower risk of 30-day and 1-year mortality with an incremental benefit observed with increasing age, as patients aged 85+ had the highest associated relative risk reductions in 30-day and 1-year mortality. In another observational study from GWTG-HF among patients with HFrEF and age ≥65 years, Greene and colleagues[33] evaluated the comparative effectiveness of angiotensin receptor blockers/neprilysin inhibitors (ARNI) therapy after discharge. They found that only 10.9% of eligible patients were prescribed ARNI at discharge, and among those who were not prescribed an ARNI, 62.0% were prescribed an ACEi/ARB. Compared to patients prescribed ACEI/ARB therapy, prescription of ARNI at the time of hospital discharge was independently associated with a significant 12-month all-cause mortality, but not all-cause or HF hospitalization.

Sodium-Glucose Cotransporter-2 Inhibitors

SGLT-2 inhibitors were found to reduce the risk of cardiovascular death and HF hospitalizations in HFrEF and are the latest addition to GDMT in HFrEF. A post hoc analysis of the DAPA-HF (Dapagliflozin and Prevention of Adverse Outcomes in Heart Failure) trial,[34] which originally evaluated the efficacy of dapagliflozin in patients with HFrEF, assessed the efficacy of the drug in attenuating adverse events stratified by frailty indices. The frailty index in this trial was measured using the Rockwood deficit accumulation approach and patients were classified as low frailty (50.4%), intermediate frailty (33.9%), and high frailty (15.7%). Background therapy was comparable across the three subgroups, with ACE/ARB/ARNI (91%), beta-blocker (95%), and MRA (63%) in the high frailty subgroup. Over a median of 18 months, there was a consistent decrease in the composite primary endpoint of worsening HF events or cardiovascular death compared to placebo, with a higher magnitude observed in the high frailty group (difference in event rate per 100 person-years in high frailty −7.9 [-13.9 to −1.9], intermediate frailty −3.2 [-6.3 to −0.2], and low frailty −3.5 [-5.7 to −1.2]). A similar trend was observed in secondary outcomes of CV death and HF hospitalizations, total HF hospitalizations, and total CV deaths. However, a significantly higher proportion of highly frail participants discontinued the treatment drug due to adverse effects including volume depletion, adverse renal event, or discontinued due to any reason.

Physical Rehabilitation

Physical limitation is prevalent in HFrEF due to older age, increasing dyspnea, fatigue, and weight gain, which leads to the worsening of frailty. In an analysis from the FRAGILE-HF study,[35] low physical performance determined by gait speed, chair stand test, and balance testing, was prevalent in approximately 85% of ambulatory chronic HF patients (both HFrEF and HFpEF) aged > 65 years, leading to reduced exercise capacity. Similarly, a post hoc analysis of the REHAB-HF trial[36] in patients aged > 65 years hospitalized for acute HF reported the presence of frailty in approximately 50% of patients on formal assessment using the Fried criteria. Additionally, a high number of patients were found to have cognitive impairment and QoL measures. However, the persistence of physical inactivity in frail patients may lead to worsening outcomes, with rehabilitation and aerobic exercise in frail patients has demonstrated improved health status. The main HF-ACTION trial[37] that evaluated aerobic exercise testing in outpatients with stable chronic HFrEF reported no significant benefit with aerobic exercise without adjustment for variables highly predictive for the primary endpoint. A post hoc analysis of the HF-ACTION trial[3] evaluated the efficacy of aerobic exercise in 2,130 patients with HFrEF stratified by frailty. Frailty was assessed using the Rockwood deficit accumulation approach and stratified categorically into frail and non-frail based on frailty indices. Over a median follow-up of approximately 3 years, a significant reduction in the composite end point of all-cause mortality and all-cause hospitalization was reported in the frail group (HR 0.83; 95% CI, 0.72–0.95) driven majorly by a reduction in all-cause hospitalizations. Meanwhile, no significant difference in the composite endpoint was noted in the non-frail group. A significant improvement in KCCQ-CSS scores was observed in both the frail and non-frail groups.

The REHAB-HF trial[38] evaluated the efficacy of a physical rehabilitation program in 349 elderly patients (mean age 73 ± 8 years) hospitalized for acute HF, specifically those that were ambulatory and functionally independent at baseline before hospitalization. Rehabilitation focused on strength, balance, mobility, and endurance exercises and was initiated in the hospital and continued outpatient, with a change in SPPB score from baseline at 3 months being the primary endpoint. The study found a significant increase in SPPB score with rehabilitation (mean between-group difference, 1.5; 95% CI, 0.9–2.0; P < 0.001). The results were unchanged when adjusted for peripheral artery disease and diabetes, and no significant difference was observed in the primary endpoint between HFrEF and HFpEF. A significant improvement in depression and KCCQ-CSS scores was observed in the intervention arm, although no change in other secondary end points e.g., all-cause mortality and hospitalizations, was reported in the intervention group. In a prespecified analysis of this trial, Pandey and colleagues[39] evaluated the effect of frailty, assessed using the modified Fried criteria, on the benefits of physical rehabilitation in this cohort (almost half had HFrEF). Frail patients were 2.6 times more likely to benefit from the intervention compared to pre-frail patients. It may seem counterintuitive but physical rehabilitation appears to improve functional limitations and quality of life in frail HF patients.

A MULTI-DOMAIN APPROACH TO FRAILTY IN HEART FAILURE

Given the evidence discussed above regarding the sustained efficacy of HFrEF therapies in frail patients, the implementation is still restricted due to clinical inertia and a heightened perceived risk of harm leading to the undertreatment of this high-risk group. It is important to note that the relationship between HFrEF and frailty is bidirectional as worsening HF leads to frailty which further imposes functional limitations leading to increased risk of worsening HF. One of the reasons why frail HF patients may perform worse than non-frail patients is likely due to the lack of adoption of comprehensive GDMT, as reported in the *post hoc* analysis of the GUIDE-IT trial.[20] Moreover, cardiac rehabilitation appears to offer heightened benefits among frail patients with HF as compared with non-frail patients. Hence it is imperative for frail patients to continue therapies to improve outcomes. Across all 4 pillars of guideline-directed medical therapy for HFrEF, in general, rates of adverse events and drug discontinuation are not significantly different between active therapy and placebo, even among patients with advanced age and frailty where drug intolerance is often of greatest concern. Simultaneous with reassuring safety across the spectrum of frailty, the totality of evidence suggests that the relative benefits of GDMT extend across the spectrum of age and frailty. However, due to the higher underlying background risk, in many cases, absolute risk reductions are greatest among older, frail, and multimorbid patients. Thus, while the risk of adverse events and potential intolerance is often emphasized by clinicians and patients when

HFrEF & Frailty

Baseline Characteristics

➢ More likely women

➢ High clinical co-morbidity burden

➢ Old age

➢ Sarcopenia

➢ Cognitive dysfunction

➢ Nutritional deficiencies

➢ Physical limitations

Outcomes

➢ Less likely to be on guideline-directed medical therapy (GDMT)

➢ Less likely to undergo cardiac rehabilitation

➢ Low health-related quality of life

➢ High symptomatic burden

➢ Increased risk of worsening heart failure events

➢ Increased risk of death

Potential Interventions

➢ Targeted strategies to improve implementation of GDMT among patients with HFrEF and comorbid frailty

➢ Specialized cardiac rehabilitation programs

➢ Management of nutritional deficiencies and cognitive impairment

➢ Multidisciplinary care with a focus on improvement in quality of life

Fig. 1. Baseline characteristics, outcomes, and potential interventions in patients with heart failure with reduced ejection (HFrEF) and frailty.

considering therapy, the "risks of omission" need to be heavily considered when deferring a trial of medical therapy among eligible patients with HFrEF and comorbid frailty, including the excess risk of death, hospitalization, and worsening quality of life. In combination with efforts to maximize the appropriate use of GDMT in this high-risk cohort, a multi-disciplinary approach should be instituted toward the care of frail HFrEF patients with a special focus on participation in cardiac rehabilitation programs. Moreover, nutritional deficiencies and cognitive impairment are common among these patients and need to be addressed. Interventions should be focused toward improving symptom burden and quality of life, in addition to an alleviation of clinically significant events e.g., hospitalizations or death (**Fig. 1**).

SUMMARY

Patients with HFrEF and comorbid frailty are a vulnerable group that are at increased risk of adverse clinical events. Some of these risks may be mitigated by the optimal implementation of beneficial therapies; however, clinical inertia hinders the implementation of medical therapies and other evidence-based management strategies, largely due to perceptions of therapeutic futility and/or risk of medication-related adverse events or intolerance. A multi-disciplinary approach with close follow-up for the repeat assessment of clinical status is required for frail HFrEF patients to address medical management, functional limitations, nutritional deficiencies, and cognitive impairment to achieve a better quality of life and event-free survival.

CLINICS CARE POINTS

- Frail HFrEF patients are more likely to be older, women, sarcopenic, nutritionally deficient, and have more cardiovascular and non-cardiovascular co-morbidities.

- Frail HFrEF patients are at up to 2-fold increased risk of mortality and all-cause hospitalizations compared to non-frail HFrEF patients.

- Frail HFrEF patients are less likely to receive comprehensive GDMT due to perceptions of therapeutic futility and/or risk of medication related adverse events or intolerance. However, GDMT is equally efficacious and safe in frail patients compared to non-frail patients based on post hoc analysis from randomized trials.

- Exercise rehabilitation is also equally efficacious in both frail and non-frail HFrEF patients.

FINANCIAL DISCLOSURES

Dr S.J. Greene has received research support from the American Heart Association, United States, Amgen, United States, AstraZeneca, United Kingdom, Bristol Myers Squibb, United States, Cytokinetics, United States, Merck, United States, Novartis, Switzerland, Pfizer, United States, and Sanofi, United States; has served on advisory boards for Amgen, AstraZeneca, Bristol Myers Squibb, Cytokinetics, and Sanofi; and has served as a consultant for Amgen, Bayer, Bristol Myers Squibb, Merck, Sanofi, and Vifor. Dr J. Butler reports personal consulting fees from Abbott, Adrenomed, Amgen, Applied Therapeutics, Array, AstraZeneca, Bayer, Boehringer Ingelheim, CVRx, G3 Pharma, Impulse Dynamics, Innolife, Janssen, LivaNova, Luitpold, Medtronic, Merck, Novartis, Novo Nordisk, Relypsa, Sequana Medical, and Vifor Pharma; and payment for lectures, presentations, speakers' bureaus, article writing or educational events from AstraZeneca, BI-Lilly, Janssen, and Novartis. Dr K.M. Talha and Dr M.S. Khan have no financial disclosures.

REFERENCES

1. Pandey A, Kitzman D, Reeves G. Frailty is intertwined with heart failure: mechanisms, prevalence, prognosis, assessment, and management. JACC Heart Fail 2019;7:1001.
2. Dewan P, Jackson A, Jhund PS, et al. The prevalence and importance of frailty in heart failure with reduced ejection fraction – an analysis of PARADIGM-HF and ATMOSPHERE. Eur J Heart Fail 2020;22:2123–33.
3. Pandey A, Segar MW, Singh S, et al. Frailty status modifies the efficacy of exercise training among patients with chronic heart failure and reduced ejection fraction: an analysis from the HF-ACTION trial. Circulation 2022;146:80–90.
4. Yang X, Lupón J, Vidán MT, et al. Impact of frailty on mortality and hospitalization in chronic heart failure: a systematic review and meta-analysis. J Am Heart Assoc 2018;7:e008251.
5. Murphy SP, Kakkar R, McCarthy CP, et al. Inflammation in heart failure: JACC state-of-the-art review. J Am Coll Cardiol 2020;75:1324–40.
6. Afilalo J, Alexander KP, Mack MJ, et al. Frailty assessment in the cardiovascular care of older adults. J Am Coll Cardiol 2014;63:747–62.
7. Kalogeropoulos A, Georgiopoulou V, Psaty BM, et al. Inflammatory markers and incident heart failure risk

in older adults: the health ABC (health, aging, and body composition) study. J Am Coll Cardiol 2010; 55:2129–37.

8. Povar-Echeverría M, Auquilla-Clavijo PE, Andrès E, et al. Interleukin-6 could be a potential prognostic factor in ambulatory elderly patients with stable heart failure: results from a pilot study. J Clin Med 2021;10:1–11.

9. van Tassell BW, Canada J, Carbone S, et al. Interleukin-1 blockade in recently decompensated systolic heart failure: results from REDHART (recently decompensated heart failure anakinra response trial). *Circ Heart Fail* 2017;10:e004373.

10. von Haehling S, Garfias Macedo T, Valentova M, et al. Muscle wasting as an independent predictor of survival in patients with chronic heart failure. J Cachexia Sarcopenia Muscle 2020;11:1242–9.

11. Buta BJ, Walston JD, Godino JG, et al. Frailty assessment instruments: systematic characterization of the uses and contexts of highly-cited instruments. Ageing Res Rev 2016;26:53.

12. Fried LP, Tangen CM, Walston J, et al. Frailty in older adults: evidence for a phenotype. *J Gerontol A Biol Sci Med Sci* 2001;56:M146–56.

13. Saum KU, Müller H, Stegmaier C, et al. Development and evaluation of a modification of the fried frailty criteria using population-independent cutpoints. J Am Geriatr Soc 2012;60:2110–5.

14. Rockwood K, Song X, MacKnight C, et al. A global clinical measure of fitness and frailty in elderly people. CMAJ (Can Med Assoc J) : Canadian Medical Association Journal 2005;173:489.

15. Searle SD, Mitnitski A, Gahbauer EA, et al. A standard procedure for creating a frailty index. BMC Geriatr 2008;8:1–10.

16. Davis MR, Lee CS, Corcoran A, et al. Gender differences in the prevalence of frailty in heart failure: a systematic review and meta-analysis. Int J Cardiol 2021;333:133–40.

17. Vidán MT, Blaya-Novakova V, Sánchez E, et al. Prevalence and prognostic impact of frailty and its components in non-dependent elderly patients with heart failure. Eur J Heart Fail 2016;18:869–75.

18. Pandey A, Group LAR, Khan MS, et al. Association of baseline and longitudinal changes in frailty burden and risk of heart failure in type 2 diabetes—findings from the look AHEAD trial. J Gerontol: Series A 2022;2022:1–9.

19. Sze S, Pellicori P, Zhang J, et al. Effect of frailty on treatment, hospitalisation and death in patients with chronic heart failure. Clin Res Cardiol 2021; 110:1249–58.

20. Khan MS, Segar MW, Usman MS, et al. Frailty, guideline-directed medical therapy, and outcomes in HFrEF: from the GUIDE-IT trial. JACC Heart Fail 2022;10:266–75.

21. Ahmed A. Digoxin and reduction in mortality and hospitalization in geriatric heart failure: importance of low doses and low serum concentrations. J Gerontol A Biol Sci Med Sci 2007;62:323.

22. Packer M, Coats AJS, Fowler MB, et al. Effect of carvedilol on survival in severe chronic heart failure. N Engl J Med 2001;344:1651–8.

23. Deedwania PC, Group for the M-HS, Gottlieb S, et al. Efficacy, safety and tolerability of β-adrenergic blockade with metoprolol CR/XL in elderly patients with heart failure. Eur Heart J 2004;25:1300–9.

24. Erland E, Philippe L, Patricia V, et al. Results from post-hoc analyses of the CIBIS II trial: effect of bisoprolol in high-risk patient groups with chronic heart failure. Eur J Heart Fail 2001;3:469–79.

25. Hernandez AF, Hammill BG, O'Connor CM, et al. Clinical effectiveness of beta-blockers in heart failure: findings from the OPTIMIZE-HF (organized program to initiate lifesaving treatment in hospitalized patients with heart failure) registry. J Am Coll Cardiol 2009;53:184–92.

26. Pitt B, Zannad F, Remme WJ, et al. The effect of spironolactone on morbidity and mortality in patients with severe heart failure. N Engl J Med 1999;341: 709–17.

27. Pitt B, Remme W, Zannad F, et al. Eplerenone, a selective aldosterone blocker, in patients with left ventricular dysfunction after myocardial infarction. *New Eng J Med*, 348, 2003,1309–1321.

28. Zannad F, McMurray JJV, Krum H, et al. Eplerenone in patients with systolic heart failure and mild symptoms. N Engl J Med 2011;364:11–21.

29. Japp D, Shah A, Fisken S, et al. Mineralocorticoid receptor antagonists in elderly patients with heart failure: a systematic review and meta-analysis. Age Ageing 2017;46:18–25.

30. Yaku H, Kato T, Morimoto T, et al. Association of mineralocorticoid receptor antagonist use with all-cause mortality and hospital readmission in older adults with acute decompensated heart failure. JAMA Netw Open 2019;2:e195892.

31. Flather MD, Yusuf S, Kober L, et al. Long-term ACE-inhibitor therapy in patients with heart failure or left-ventricular dysfunction: a systematic overview of data from individual patients. *Lancet* 2000;355: 1575–81.

32. Gilstrap L, Solomon N, Chiswell K, et al. The association between beta-blocker and renin angiotensin system inhibitor use after HFrEF hospitalization and outcomes in older patients. J Card Fail 2022.

33. Greene SJ, Choi S, Lippmann SJ, et al. Clinical effectiveness of sacubitril/valsartan among patients hospitalized for heart failure with reduced ejection fraction. Journal of the American Heart Association J Am Heart Assoc 2021;10:21459.

34. Butt JH, Dewan P, Merkely B, et al. Efficacy and safety of dapagliflozin according to frailty in heart failure with reduced ejection fraction. Ann Intern Med 2022;175:820–30.

35. Saka K, Konishi M, Kagiyama N, et al. Impact of physical performance on exercise capacity in older patients with heart failure with reduced and preserved ejection fraction. Exp Gerontol 2021;156:111626.

36. Warraich HJ, Kitzman DW, Whellan DJ, et al. Physical function, frailty, cognition, depression, and quality of life in hospitalized adults ≥60 years with acute decompensated heart failure with preserved versus reduced ejection fraction. Circ Heart Fail 2018;11:e005254.

37. O'Connor CM, Whellan DJ, Lee KL, et al. Efficacy and safety of exercise training in patients with chronic heart failure: HF-ACTION randomized controlled trial. JAMA 2009;301:1439–50.

38. Kitzman DW, Whellan DJ, Duncan P, et al. Physical rehabilitation for older patients hospitalized for heart failure. N Engl J Med 2021;385:203–16.

39. Pandey A, Kitzman DW, Nelson MB, et al. Frailty and effects of a multidomain physical rehabilitation intervention among older patients hospitalized for acute heart failure: a secondary analysis of a randomized clinical trial. JAMA Cardiol 2023;8(2):167–76.

Obesity in Heart Failure with Reduced Ejection Fraction
Time to Address the Elephant in the Room

Matthew B. Amdahl, MD, PhD[a], Varun Sundaram, MBBS[b],
Yogesh N.V. Reddy, MBBS[a,c],*

KEYWORDS

- HFrEF • Heart failure • Obesity • Weight loss

KEY POINTS

- Obesity is an important comorbidity to manage in patients with heart failure with reduced ejection fraction (HFrEF) with important associations with atrial fibrillation, adverse hemodynamics, and poor functional status.
- Although a statistical obesity paradox has been observed where obesity in HFrEF is associated with better outcomes, there is no evidence that intentional weight loss is harmful in HFrEF.
- Randomized trials testing intentional weight loss are needed in obese HFrEF patients.

INTRODUCTION

The prevalence of obesity is rapidly increasing in the Western World, and by 2030, it is estimated that one out of two adults in the United States will be obese.[1] Obesity is clearly linked to incident heart failure,[2] and therefore, the prevalence of heart failure is expected to exponentially increase. Although obesity seems to be associated with both heart failure with preserved ejection fraction (HFpEF) and reduced ejection fraction (HFrEF),[3] the association between obesity and HFpEF seems to be stronger[3,4] along with clear biological demonstration of an obese HFpEF phenotype.[5–7] Subclinical abnormalities in myocardial mechanics are present in obese patients with preclinical HFpEF further supporting a causal relationship with HFpEF.[8–10] However, the causal relationship and clinical implications of obesity in patients with a dilated cardiomyopathy and HFrEF are less clear. In this review, the authors summarize the evidence and potential implications of obesity in patients with a dilated cardiomyopathy and HFrEF.

CHALLENGES WITH DEFINITIONS OF OBESITY IN HEART FAILURE WITH REDUCED EJECTION FRACTION

Obesity is pragmatically defined based on an individual's overall weight for a given height as the body mass index (BMI) (ie, weight/height^2). Although this is easy to calculate and generally correlates with excess adiposity, there may be vastly different distributions of fat mass for any BMI. Therefore, for the same BMI, one individual may have increased muscle mass, whereas another individual may have more visceral or subcutaneous adiposity contributing to heterogeneity across disease states for the implications of BMI on outcomes. In HFrEF specifically, with disease progression, there is systemic inflammation and

[a] Department of Cardiovascular Diseases, Mayo Clinic, 200 1st Street Southwest, Rochester, MN 55905, USA;
[b] Louis Stokes Cleveland VA Medical Center, Case Western Reserve University, 10701 East Blvd, Cleveland, OH 44106, USA; [c] University Hospitals Medical Center, Cleveland, OH, USA
* Corresponding author.
E-mail address: reddy.yogesh@mayo.edu

0733-8651/23/© 2023 Elsevier Inc. All rights reserved.

gut congestion with cardiac cachexia and pro-gressive loss of lean muscle mass.[11] Depending on baseline BMI before the development of wors-ening HFrEF, there is therefore tremendous het-erogeneity in body composition as HFrEF progresses and BMI changes generally better reflect changes in lean body mass in patients with HFrEF.[12]

CAN OBESITY CAUSE HEART FAILURE WITH REDUCED EJECTION FRACTION?

Although obesity is well established as a causal factor for the development of heart failure,[2] recent data have suggested that the link between obesity is stronger for HFpEF[3] with the identification of a clear phenotype of obese HFpEF.[3–7] In contrast, the association between obesity and HFrEF is less robust compared with HFpEF[3] and not univer-sally observed.[4,13] This weaker association be-tween obesity and HFrEF is further confounded by the independent role obesity exerts in causing hypertension and coronary artery disease[14] which by themselves are causal factors for clinical HFrEF. Furthermore, among patients with morbid obesity, the duration of obesity predicts incident HF but systolic dysfunction seems to be uncom-mon[15] and most patients have a phenotype with preserved systolic function with either HFpEF[6,16] or frank high output heart failure from obesity.[17] Obesity is also extremely common in the commu-nity, and only a very small minority with obesity de-velops HFrEF further arguing against a strong causal role with a likely need for individual genetic susceptibility to HFrEF for disease manifestation.

There is however emerging evidence that obesity may directly contribute to HFrEF in a sub-set of patients with nonischemic cardiomyopathy independent of coronary artery disease. Popula-tion studies from Sweden demonstrated an important but modest association between obesity in adolescence and incident HFrEF in both men and women independent of coronary disease and myocardial infarction.[18,19] Obese HFrEF patients have also been observed to have higher rates of idiopathic cardiomyopathy compared with nonobese HFrEF.[20] A carefully performed study also demonstrated differences in myocardial energetics between obese and nonobese nonischemic HFrEF, and in the obese HFrEF subset there was an improvement in myocardial remodeling and metabolic efficiency with weight loss.[21] Therefore, there is emerging evidence that obesity may directly cause noni-schemic HFrEF in an important subset of patients and this may have treatment implications, because weight loss in such subsets of patients

with "obesity related" HFrEF may be theoretically beneficial.

PATHOPHYSIOLOGY OF HEART FAILURE WITH REDUCED EJECTION FRACTION AND OBESITY

Independent of whether obesity is causal in an in-dividual patient's cardiomyopathy, there is evi-dence that obesity may affect HFrEF in numerous ways. These include (1) direct effects on hemodynamics, (2) activation or suppression of numerous signaling pathways, (3) alteration of myocardial energetics/metabolism, and (4) driving specific patterns of cardiac remodeling.

Hemodynamics

Obesity is well-known to have numerous effects on hemodynamics,[22] both direct and indirect, which may modulate the phenotype of HFrEF. Obesity is associated with an increased blood volume and venous return,[23] which in function-ally normal hearts results in an abnormal in-crease in cardiac output with increased LV (left ventricle) stroke work. In its most extreme form, this can result in high output heart failure,[17] but in patients with inherent abnormal myocardial remodeling and HFrEF, the increased volume load exacerbates the increase in left and right-sided filling pressures.[20] In HFrEF hearts with dilated cardiomyopathy, an increase in venous return often decreases cardiac output and stroke volume despite increases in biventricular filling pressures due to the phenomenon of relative pericardial restraint and constriction like physi-ology.[24] An increase in heart size in dilated car-diomyopathy results in a stretch in the native pericardium with resultant compressive contact force on the heart which increases intracardiac filling pressures while at the same time decreasing LV preload due to the extrinsic compressive restraint.[25] Obesity has been clearly associated with worse pericardial re-straint in obese HFpEF,[6] and with pericardial re-straint being common in dilated cardiomyopathy of all types, it is likely that comorbid obesity also worsens pericardial restraint and associated he-modynamics in HFrEF. Obesity may also variably affect arterial afterload depending on fat distribu-tion with an increase in central vascular stiffness (with visceral adiposity) or decrease in systemic vascular resistance (with greater subcutaneous adiposity).[26] One study specifically examined patients with obesity and dilated cardiomyopa-thy with mean left ventricular ejection fraction (LVEF) of 25% in the obese group and found that obese HFrEF patients had higher left- and right-sided filling pressures and pulmonary artery pressures which were all associated with the magnitude of obesity.[20]

Adipokines and Altered Signaling

In addition to direct hemodynamic effects, obesity may impact numerous signaling pathways relevant to HFrEF. One major mechanism is secretion of various mediators by adipocytes, which are broadly referred to as adipokines. Many adipokines, including IL (interleukin)-1β, IL-6, and resistin, are markedly pro-inflammatory and are thought to drive numerous deleterious pathways including chronic oxidative stress, neurohormonal overactivity, and impair myocardial performance.[27] There is also significant activation of the renin/angiotensin/aldosterone system in obesity through mechanisms including angiotensinogen production by adipocytes,[28] stimulation of the sympathetic nervous system via leptin secretion,[29] and direct compression of renal vasculature by adipose tissue.[30] Obesity also results in elevated tissue neprilysin activity that increases degradation of natriuretic peptides with increase in adverse cardiac remodeling.[31] Obesity also causes a downregulation of adiponectin, a molecule primarily made by adipocytes that has been shown to exert numerous beneficial effects in heart failure,[32] and obese HFrEF patients further demonstrate adiponectin resistance at the receptor level.[33]

Energetics and Metabolism

The heart in obese patients even without heart failure demonstrates energetic abnormalities associated with abnormally increased resting adenosine triphosphate (ATP) demand through creatine kinase, with inability to further increase ATP delivery with exertion, and these changes are reversible with weight loss.[34] In patients with obese compared with nonobese HFrEF, there is an abnormally increased resting ATP demand through creatine kinase with a decrease in ATP delivery during exertion, and these changes were reversible with weight loss with improved ejection fraction and myocardial remodeling.[21] In contrast to the failing heart which attempts to shift from fatty acid to glucose metabolism,[35] obesity is associated with increased fatty acid uptake and utilization[36] and through accompanying insulin resistance, limits the ability of myocardium to increase glucose utilization during periods of increased energy demand.[35,37] In severe obesity, there is also thought to be increased uncoupling of the mitochondrial electron transport chain,[38] further reducing energetic efficiency.

Remodeling

Through the mechanisms detailed above, obesity may independently impact cardiac remodeling regardless of etiology of underlying HFrEF. Obesity can result in a variable myocardial remodeling pattern but often causes concentric hypertrophy regardless of blood pressure.[39] Myocardial biopsies of obese HFrEF patients have been found to show high rates (67%) of myocyte hypertrophy.[20] Obesity is also strongly associated with adverse right heart remodeling and abnormal right ventricular pulmonary artery coupling[40,15] and there seems to be improvement with weight loss.[41] Obesity is also a risk factor for incident atrial fibrillation in HFrEF[42] and likely directly impacts left atrial remodeling[15] as a mediator of atrial fibrillation risk.

IMPACT OF OBESITY ON SYMPTOMS IN HEART FAILURE WITH REDUCED EJECTION FRACTION

Obesity has also been shown to influence symptom character and severity in HFrEF patients (**Fig. 1**). By body composition or BMI, obese patients have been found to have worse New York Heart Association (NYHA) functional class[12] and shorter 6-minute walk distance compared with their nonobese counterparts.[21] Obese patients with HFrEF also have poorer health-related quality of life and worse depression scores[43] and this is similar to that of patients with obese HFpEF.[5]

OBESITY AND ITS ASSOCIATION WITH OUTCOMES IN HEART FAILURE WITH REDUCED EJECTION FRACTION: THE MISLEADING STATISTICAL OBESITY PARADOX

One consistent and overinterpreted observation in HFrEF is the so-called "Obesity Paradox," in which obese patients with HFrEF have been shown in numerous studies to have improved survival compared with underweight and normal weight patients.[44–46] Although numerous scientific hypotheses have been put forward to explain why obesity may be protective and beneficial in HFrEF, there is no randomized trial evidence to support that intentional weight gain to achieve overweight or obese status in HFrEF is beneficial. The obesity paradox has been observed in a myriad of disease states across cardiology and medicine with no unifying pathophysiological bases including heart failure, cancer, myocardial infarction, pulmonary arterial hypertension, and atrial fibrillation among others[47–49] and is therefore most likely a complex statistical bias in the analysis of association

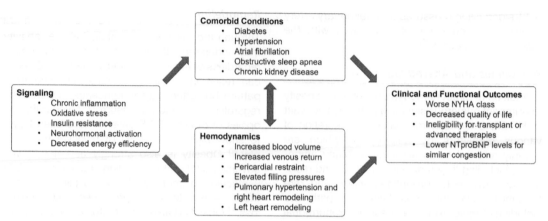

Fig. 1. Impact of obesity on heart failure with reduced ejection fraction. NTproBNP, N terminal prohormone of brain natriuretic peptide.

between BMI and mortality that exists regardless of disease state. Unintentional weight loss in HFrEF is a marker of worsening heart failure with increased mortality[50] and is likely an important contributor to the observed association between lower BMI and worse outcomes. Such reverse causation and unmeasured confounding coupled with collider stratification bias likely all contribute to the obesity paradox along with the fact that BMI poorly reflects lean muscle mass changes in HFrEF. There is therefore currently no evidence-based reason to avoid healthy intentional weight loss in obese HFrEF patients and certainly no randomized evidence to support an intentional increase in weight to the overweight or obese range in HFrEF.

TREATMENT IMPLICATIONS OF OBESITY IN HEART FAILURE WITH REDUCED EJECTION FRACTION
Weight loss

Weight loss has demonstrated a strong protective effect in observational studies to prevent future heart failure events,[51,52] although whether HFrEF specifically is prevented is unclear as there is stronger biological rationale for weight loss to prevent incident HFpEF.[53] Ultimately, a key determinant of the benefit (or harm) associated with weight loss in HFrEF is the intentionality of weight loss. Unintentional weight loss, in the form of wasting or cachexia, is known to be a very poor prognostic factor in patients with previously normal weight.[50] Intentional weight loss, on the other hand, likely has significant benefits, although this remains to be tested in a randomized trial in HFrEF. Observational studies have shown improvement in systolic function and myocardial energy efficiency with intentional

weight loss in patients with HFrEF potentially related to obesity.[21] Although most studies have achieved weight loss primarily with lifestyle interventions, bariatric surgery in small observational series has shown improvement in LVEF and dramatic weight loss without excess mortality.[54,55] There is however early procedural risk to surgical approaches to weight loss in patients with HFrEF. With the emergence of effective weight loss drugs like the glucagon-like peptide 1 (GLP-1) agonists such as semaglutide and tirzepatide,[56,57] there is increased enthusiasm that safe weight loss in obese patients can be achieved with drug therapy. Enthusiasm for use of these drugs in HFrEF patients with obesity is, however, tempered by the signal for harm observed with use of the GLP-1 agonist liraglutide in nonobese HFrEF patients where there was a signal for increased risk of heart failure hospitalization.[58] Whether this risk–benefit ratio is altered in patients with an idiopathic HFrEF phenotype with obesity remains to be determined.

SGLT2 (sodium-glucose cotransporter-2) inhibitors

SGLT2 inhibitors are known to be beneficial in HFrEF regardless of diabetes status and importantly seem to promote greater weight loss among patients with obesity.[59] This is related in part to the enhanced nutrient deprivation signaling where obesity can be considered a disorder of nutrient excess.[60] Importantly, although the SGLT2 inhibitor HFrEF trials demonstrate a similar obesity paradox as other studies, SGLT2 inhibitor-induced weight loss (which is intentional) is not associated with worse outcomes, conclusively refuting the presence of an obesity paradox.[59,61]

Mineralocorticoid receptor antagonists

Mineralocorticoid receptor antagonists are a standard part of guideline-directed medical therapy (GDMT) in all patients with HFrEF, but one trial has found that eplerenone was even more beneficial in HFrEF patients with high waist circumference than in those with a normal waist size.[62]

Angiotensin receptor blockers + neprilysin inhibitors (ARNIs)

Although combined ARB (angiotension receptor blocker) + neprilysin inhibitors are known to be beneficial in HFrEF,[63] studies examining the relationship between BMI and outcomes between these medications have thus far not found any significant variation in outcomes when patients are stratified according to BMI.[64] The subsequent analysis of the PARADIGM-HF trial, however, identified improvement in A1c in patients treated with sacubitril/valsartan versus enalapril, suggesting a possible benefit for obese patients given their elevated risk of diabetes.[65]

Continuous positive airway pressure (CPAP) in comorbid obstructive sleep apnea

There is no randomized trial evidence that treating coexisting obstructive sleep apnea in HFrEF improves cardiovascular outcomes. In fact, a trial treating central sleep apnea in HFrEF paradoxically demonstrated increased mortality with this approach.[66] Therefore, healthy weight loss and optimization of underlying heart failure should be actively encouraged to improve sleep apnea in HFrEF.

Atrial fibrillation

Obesity is associated with incident atrial fibrillation in HFrEF.[42] Although there are no randomized trials testing weight loss to improve atrial fibrillation in HFrEF, a randomized trial in obese patients with atrial fibrillation demonstrated decreased recurrence rates with healthy weight loss.[67] Therefore, treatment of obesity even in HFrEF may improve atrial fibrillation, although this requires dedicated trials in HFrEF.

- Advanced heart failure

Severe obesity in HFrEF is generally considered a contraindication to transplantation and therefore has important treatment implications in advanced heart failure. Observational series have supported the use of bariatric surgery with left ventricular assist device (LVAD) implantation as well as use of these therapies to improve obesity to eventually receive heart transplantation.[68,69]

CLINICS CARE POINTS

- Obese patients are at higher risk for the development of heart failure with reduced ejection fraction. There are emerging data that a subset of nonischemic heart failure with reduced ejection fraction (HFrEF) patients may have their disease driven primarily by obesity. In HFrEF patients with other etiologies, obesity may be an important comorbidity with clinical implications.

- Obese patients who develop HFrEF often have worse symptoms, functional status, energetics, and hemodynamics.

- The obesity paradox of improved survival at higher body mass index is a statistical artifact and healthy weight loss is likely safe in obese HFrEF, although it has not yet been tested in randomized trials.

DISCLOSURE

The authors have nothing to disclose.

FUNDING

VS is supported by grants from Care Source Research Foundation. YNR is supported by National Heart, Lung, And Blood Institute of the National Institutes of Health (NHLBI) Award Number K23HL164901, grants from Sleep Number, Bayer, United pharmaceuticals, and the Earl Wood Career Development Award from Mayo Clinic.

REFERENCES

1. Ward ZJ, Bleich SN, Cradock AL, et al. Projected U.S. state-level prevalence of adult obesity and severe obesity. N Engl J Med 2019;381(25):2440–50.
2. Kenchaiah S, Evans JC, Levy D, et al. Obesity and the risk of heart failure. N Engl J Med 2002;347(5): 305–13.
3. Savji N, Meijers WC, Bartz TM, et al. The association of obesity and cardiometabolic traits with incident HFpEF and HFrEF. JACC Heart Fail 2018;6(8):701–9.
4. Pandey A, LaMonte M, Klein L, et al. Relationship between physical activity, body mass index, and risk of heart failure. J Am Coll Cardiol 2017;69(9): 1129–42.
5. Reddy YNV, Rikhi A, Obokata M, et al. Quality of life in heart failure with preserved ejection fraction: importance of obesity, functional capacity, and physical inactivity. Eur J Heart Fail 2020;22(6): 1009–18.

6. Obokata M, Reddy YNV, Pislaru SV, et al. Evidence supporting the existence of a distinct obese phenotype of heart failure with preserved ejection fraction. Circulation 2017;136(1):6–19.

7. Reddy YNV, Lewis GD, Shah SJ, et al. Characterization of the obese phenotype of heart failure with preserved ejection fraction: a RELAX trial ancillary study. Mayo Clin Proc 2019;94(7):1199–209.

8. Stoddard MF, Tseuda K, Thomas M, et al. The influence of obesity on left ventricular filling and systolic function. Am Heart J 1992;124(3):694–9.

9. Garg PK, Biggs ML, Kizer JR, et al. Associations of body size and composition with subclinical cardiac dysfunction in older individuals: the cardiovascular health study. Int J Obes 2021;45(12):2539–45.

10. Selvaraj S, Martinez EE, Aguilar FG, et al. Association of central adiposity with adverse cardiac mechanics: findings from the hypertension genetic epidemiology network study. Circ Cardiovasc Imaging 2016;9(6):e004396.

11. Zhao SP, Zeng LH. Elevated plasma levels of tumor necrosis factor in chronic heart failure with cachexia. Int J Cardiol 1997;58(3):257–61.

12. Oreopoulos A, Ezekowitz JA, McAlister FA, et al. Association between direct measures of body composition and prognostic factors in chronic heart failure. Mayo Clin Proc 2010;85(7):609–17.

13. Rao VN, Zhao D, Allison MA, et al. Adiposity and incident heart failure and its subtypes: MESA (multi-ethnic study of atherosclerosis). JACC Heart Fail 2018;6(12):999–1007.

14. Kim MS, Kim WJ, Khera AV, et al. Association between adiposity and cardiovascular outcomes: an umbrella review and meta-analysis of observational and Mendelian randomization studies. Eur Heart J 2021;42(34):3388–403.

15. Alpert MA, Terry BE, Mulekar M, et al. Cardiac morphology and left ventricular function in normotensive morbidly obese patients with and without congestive heart failure, and effect of weight loss. Am J Cardiol 1997;80(6):736–40.

16. Reddy YNV, Carter RE, Obokata M, et al. A simple, evidence-based approach to help guide diagnosis of heart failure with preserved ejection fraction. Circulation 2018;138(9):861–70.

17. Reddy YNV, Melenovsky V, Redfield MM, et al. High-output heart failure: a 15-year experience. J Am Coll Cardiol 2016;68(5):473–82.

18. Robertson J, Lindgren M, Schaufelberger M, et al. Body mass index in young women and risk of cardiomyopathy: a long-term follow-up study in Sweden. Circulation 2020;141(7):520–9.

19. Robertson J, Schaufelberger M, Lindgren M, et al. Higher body mass index in adolescence predicts cardiomyopathy risk in midlife. Circulation 2019;140(2):117–25.

20. Kasper EK, Hruban RH, Baughman KL. Cardiomyopathy of obesity: a clinicopathologic evaluation of 43 obese patients with heart failure. Am J Cardiol 1992;70(9):921–4.

21. Rayner JJ, Peterzan MA, Clarke WT, et al. Obesity modifies the energetic phenotype of dilated cardiomyopathy. Eur Heart J 2021;43(9):868–77.

22. Reddy YNV, Anantha-Narayanan M, Obokata M, et al. Hemodynamic effects of weight loss in obesity: a systematic review and meta-analysis. JACC Heart Fail 2019;7(8):678–87.

23. Alexander JK, Dennis EW, Smith WG, et al. Blood volume, cardiac output, and distribution of systemic blood flow in extreme obesity. Cardiovasc Res Cent Bull 1962;1:39–44.

24. Borlaug BA, Reddy YNV. The role of the pericardium in heart failure: implications for pathophysiology and treatment. JACC Heart Fail 2019;7(7):574–85.

25. Atherton JJ, Moore TD, Lele SS, et al. Diastolic ventricular interaction in chronic heart failure. Lancet Lond Engl 1997;349(9067):1720–4.

26. Neeland IJ, Gupta S, Ayers CR, et al. Relation of regional fat distribution to left ventricular structure and function. Circ Cardiovasc Imaging 2013;6(5):800–7.

27. Hofmann U, Heuer S, Meder K, et al. The proinflammatory cytokines TNF-α and IL-1β impair economy of contraction in human myocardium. Cytokine 2007;39(3):157–62.

28. Ailhaud G, Fukamizu A, Massiera F, et al. Angiotensinogen, angiotensin II and adipose tissue development. Int J Obes 2000;24(S4):S33–5.

29. Sharma AM. Is There a rationale for angiotensin blockade in the management of obesity hypertension? Hypertension 2004;44(1):12–9.

30. Hall JE, do Carmo JM, da Silva AA, et al. Obesity-induced hypertension: interaction of neurohumoral and renal mechanisms. Circ Res 2015;116(6):991–1006.

31. Standeven KF, Hess K, Carter AM, et al. Neprilysin, obesity and the metabolic syndrome. Int J Obes 2011;35(8):1031–40.

32. Packer M. Leptin-aldosterone-neprilysin axis: identification of its distinctive role in the pathogenesis of the three phenotypes of heart failure in people with obesity. Circulation 2018;137(15):1614–31.

33. Van Berendoncks AM, Garnier A, Beckers P, et al. Functional adiponectin resistance at the level of the skeletal muscle in mild to moderate chronic heart failure. Circ Heart Fail 2010;3(2):185–94.

34. Rayner JJ, Peterzan MA, Watson WD, et al. Myocardial energetics in obesity: enhanced ATP delivery through creatine kinase with blunted stress response. Circulation 2020;141(14):1152–63.

35. Neglia D, De Caterina A, Marraccini P, et al. Impaired myocardial metabolic reserve and

substrate selection flexibility during stress in patients with idiopathic dilated cardiomyopathy. Am J Physiol Heart Circ Physiol 2007;293(6):H3270–8.

36. Rayner JJ, Banerjee R, Holloway CJ, et al. The relative contribution of metabolic and structural abnormalities to diastolic dysfunction in obesity. Int J Obes 2018;42(3):441–7.

37. Peterson LR, Herrero P, Schechtman KB, et al. Effect of obesity and insulin resistance on myocardial substrate metabolism and efficiency in young women. Circulation 2004;109(18):2191–6.

38. Ruiz-Ramírez A, López-Acosta O, Barrios-Maya MA, et al. Cell death and heart failure in obesity: role of uncoupling proteins. Oxid Med Cell Longev 2016; 2016:1–11.

39. Woodiwiss AJ, Libhaber CD, Majane OHI, et al. Obesity promotes left ventricular concentric rather than eccentric geometric remodeling and hypertrophy independent of blood pressure. Am J Hypertens 2008;21(10):1144–51.

40. Obokata M, Reddy YNV, Melenovsky V, et al. Deterioration in right ventricular structure and function over time in patients with heart failure and preserved ejection fraction. Eur Heart J 2019;40(8):689–97.

41. Sorimachi H, Obokata M, Omote K, et al. Long-term changes in cardiac structure and function following bariatric surgery. J Am Coll Cardiol 2022;80(16): 1501–12.

42. Kotecha D, Holmes J, Krum H, et al. Efficacy of β blockers in patients with heart failure plus atrial fibrillation: an individual-patient data meta-analysis. Lancet Lond Engl 2014;384(9961):2235–43.

43. Evangelista LS, Moser DK, Westlake C, et al. Impact of obesity on quality of life and depression in patients with heart failure. Eur J Heart Fail 2006;8(7):750–5.

44. Oreopoulos A, Padwal R, Kalantar-Zadeh K, et al. Body mass index and mortality in heart failure: a meta-analysis. Am Heart J 2008;156(1):13–22.

45. Ather S, Chan W, Bozkurt B, et al. Impact of noncardiac comorbidities on morbidity and mortality in a predominantly male population with heart failure and preserved versus reduced ejection fraction. J Am Coll Cardiol 2012;59(11):998–1005.

46. Lavie CJ, Alpert MA, Arena R, et al. Impact of obesity and the obesity paradox on prevalence and prognosis in heart failure. JACC Heart Fail 2013;1(2):93–102.

47. Angerås O, Albertsson P, Karason K, et al. Evidence for obesity paradox in patients with acute coronary syndromes: a report from the Swedish Coronary Angiography and Angioplasty Registry. Eur Heart J 2013;34(5):345–53.

48. Sandhu RK, Ezekowitz J, Andersson U, et al. The "obesity paradox" in atrial fibrillation: observations from the ARISTOTLE (Apixaban for reduction in stroke and other thromboembolic events in atrial fibrillation) trial. Eur Heart J 2016;37(38):2869–78.

49. Mazimba S, Holland E, Nagarajan V, et al. Obesity paradox in group 1 pulmonary hypertension: analysis of the NIH-Pulmonary hypertension registry. Int J Obes 2017;41(8):1164–8.

50. Anker SD, Ponikowski P, Varney S, et al. Wasting as independent risk factor for mortality in chronic heart failure. Lancet 1997;349(9058):1050–3.

51. Aminian A, Zajichek A, Arterburn DE, et al. Association of metabolic surgery with major adverse cardiovascular outcomes in patients with type 2 diabetes and obesity. JAMA 2019. https://doi.org/10.1001/jama.2019.14231.

52. Sundström J, Bruze G, Ottosson J, et al. Weight loss and heart failure: a nationwide study of gastric bypass surgery versus intensive lifestyle treatment. Circulation 2017;135(17):1577–85.

53. Patel KV, Bahnson JL, Gaussoin SA, et al. Association of baseline and longitudinal changes in body composition measures with risk of heart failure and myocardial infarction in type 2 diabetes: findings from the look AHEAD trial. Circulation 2020; 142(25):2420–30.

54. Vest AR, Patel P, Schauer PR, et al. Clinical and echocardiographic outcomes after bariatric surgery in obese patients with left ventricular systolic dysfunction. Circ Heart Fail 2016;9(3):e002260.

55. Shoar S, Manzoor A, Abdelrazek AS, et al. Parallel improvement of systolic function with surgical weight loss in patients with heart failure and reduced ejection fraction: a systematic review and patient-level meta-analysis. Surg Obes Relat Dis 2022;18(3): 433–8.

56. Rubino D, Abrahamsson N, Davies M, et al. Effect of continued weekly subcutaneous semaglutide vs placebo on weight loss maintenance in adults with overweight or obesity: the STEP 4 Randomized clinical trial. JAMA 2021;325(14):1414–25.

57. Jastreboff AM, Aronne LJ, Ahmad NN, et al. Tirzepatide once weekly for the treatment of obesity. N Engl J Med 2022;387(3):205–16.

58. Margulies KB, Hernandez AF, Redfield MM, et al. Effects of liraglutide on clinical stability among patients with advanced heart failure and reduced ejection fraction: a randomized clinical trial. JAMA 2016;316(5):500–8.

59. Anker SD, Khan MS, Butler J, et al. Weight change and clinical outcomes in heart failure with reduced ejection fraction: insights from EMPEROR-Reduced. Eur J Heart Fail 2023;25(1):117–27.

60. Zannad F, Ferreira JP, Butler J, et al. Effect of empagliflozin on circulating proteomics in heart failure: mechanistic insights into the EMPEROR programme. Eur Heart J 2022;43(48):4991–5002.

61. Adamson C, Jhund PS, Docherty KF, et al. Efficacy of dapagliflozin in heart failure with reduced ejection fraction according to body mass index. Eur J Heart Fail 2021;23(10):1662–72.

62. Olivier A, Pitt B, Girerd N, et al. Effect of eplerenone in patients with heart failure and reduced ejection fraction: potential effect modification by abdominal obesity. Insight from the EMPHASIS-HF trial: Abdominal adiposity as biomarker for MRA efficacy. Eur J Heart Fail 2017;19(9):1186–97.

63. McMurray JJV, Packer M, Desai AS, et al. Angiotensin–neprilysin inhibition versus enalapril in heart failure. N Engl J Med 2014;371(11):993–1004.

64. Kido K, Bianco C, Caccamo M, et al. Association of body mass index with clinical outcomes in patients with heart failure with reduced ejection fraction treated with sacubitril/valsartan. J Cardiovasc Pharmacol Ther 2021;26(6):619–24.

65. Seferovic JP, Claggett B, Seidelmann SB, et al. Effect of sacubitril/valsartan versus enalapril on glycaemic control in patients with heart failure and diabetes: a post-hoc analysis from the PARADIGM-HF trial. Lancet Diabetes Endocrinol 2017;5(5):333–40.

66. Cowie MR, Woehrle H, Wegscheider K, et al. Adaptive servo-ventilation for central sleep apnea in systolic heart failure. N Engl J Med 2015;373(12):1095–105.

67. Abed HS, Wittert GA, Leong DP, et al. Effect of weight reduction and cardiometabolic risk factor management on symptom burden and severity in patients with atrial fibrillation: a randomized clinical trial. JAMA 2013;310(19):2050–60.

68. Caceres M, Czer LSC, Esmailian F, et al. Bariatric surgery in severe obesity and end-stage heart failure with mechanical circulatory support as a bridge to successful heart transplantation: a case report. Transplant Proc 2013;45(2):798–9.

69. Lockard KL, Allen C, Lohmann D, et al. Bariatric surgery for a patient with a heartmate II ventricular assist device for destination therapy. Prog Transplant 2013;23(1):28–32.

The Uncertain Benefit from Implantable Cardioverter-Defibrillators in Nonischemic Cardiomyopathy
How to Guide Clinical Decision-Making?

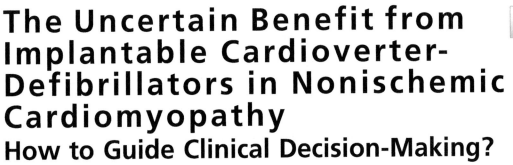

Mohsin Khan, MD, Arshad Jahangir, MD, FHRS*

KEYWORDS

- Heart failure • ICD • Sudden cardiac death • Nonischemic cardiomyopathy
- Ventricular tachycardia

KEY POINTS

- Life-threatening cardiac dysrhythmias remain a significant cause of mortality in patients with non-ischemic cardiomyopathy (NICM). The mortality benefit of implantable cardioverter-defibrillators (ICD) for the primary prevention of sudden cardiac death in patients with NICM on guideline-directed medical therapy is uncertain.
- A thorough evaluation with the incorporation of clinical, biochemical, imaging, electrical, and genetic analysis may improve the identification of high-risk patients on guideline-directed therapy who could benefit from the primary prevention of ICD implantation.

INTRODUCTION

Life-threatening cardiac dysrhythmias remain a significant cause of mortality in patients with heart failure (HF).[1] Immediate cardioversion or defibrillation by implantable cardioverter-defibrillator (ICD) has emerged as an effective therapy for reducing overall mortality in patients who have survived sudden cardiac arrest or experienced sustained ventricular arrhythmias.[2–5] In patients at high risk for sudden cardiac arrest, particularly those with severe left ventricular (LV) dysfunction and HF symptoms that persist despite optimum medical therapy, an ICD is recommended for the primary prevention of sudden cardiac death (SCD) in ischemic cardiomyopathy (ICM) and nonischemic dilated cardiomyopathy (NIDCM). Since SCD accounts for approximately one-third of the deaths in patients with NIDCM,[1,2] with an annual incidence of ~3 to 5%, and given the dread of this being the initial presentation, its prevention via the implementation of proper interventions is critical and requires the identification of high-risk individuals.[6]

The evidence for primary prevention ICD in patients with ICM is strong and comes from several randomized controlled trials (RCT).[2–5] However, data for patients with NIDCM treated with guideline-directed medical therapy (GDMT) are not as robust,[7–10] with recent studies raising questions regarding the effectiveness of ICD utilization in reducing overall mortality.[11] The sequential addition of newer pharmaceuticals and cardiac resynchronization therapy (CRT) in HF management have each contributed to a reduction in SCD and overall mortality compared with the early clinical trials assessing ICD therapy efficacy on

Aurora Cardiovascular and Thoracic Services, Center for Advanced Atrial Fibrillation Therapies, Aurora Sinai/Aurora St. Luke's Medical Centers, Advocate Aurora Health, 2801 West Kinnickinnic River Parkway, Suite 777, Milwaukee, WI 53215, USA
* Corresponding author. Aurora St. Luke's Medical Center, 2801 West Kinnickinnic River Parkway, Suite 130, Milwaukee, WI 53215.
E-mail address: wi.publishing44@aah.org

Cardiol Clin 41 (2023) 545–555
https://doi.org/10.1016/j.ccl.2023.06.005

which current recommendations are based.[3] As the competing non-arrhythmic risk of mortality increases with advancing age and associated comorbidities, the overall efficacy of ICD therapy in decreasing early mortality is reduced.[12] Pooled data from landmark ICD clinical trials show that patients with nonischemic cardiomyopathy (NICM) experience a similar risk of life-threatening ventricular arrhythmic events as patients with ICM, with non-sudden cardiac death being dominant, but they have a relatively lower risk of all-cause mortality.[13]

Current guidelines from professional societies recommend ICD implantation for the primary prevention of SCD in NIDCM,[2–5] based on a few RCTs, their pooled analysis, meta-analysis, and information from large-scale observational studies from ICD registries and population databases.[14–16] In this review, we will summarize the data, focusing on the risk of life-threatening arrhythmias with HF in NIDCM, evidence for the efficacy and safety of ICD therapy for primary prevention, and current recommendations by professional cardiac and electrophysiology societies for ICD implantation for the primary prevention of SCD in these patients.[2–5] We will also highlight data on emerging tools and technology for the identification of high-risk patients who could benefit most from a primary prevention ICD implant.

Risk of Life-Threatening Arrhythmias in Nonischemic Dilated Cardiomyopathy with Heart Failure

NIDCM is a heterogenous condition that results from a number of primary and secondary myocardial diseases and has a genetic predisposition in a substantial proportion of patients.[17] Improved insight into the pathophysiological processes underlying cardiomyopathies and their progression, the development of newer therapeutics, and the results from RCTs have allowed the advancement of medical therapies and other device-based interventions, such as the use of CRT and LV assist devices, that have further improved the outcomes of patients with NIDCM, including overall prognosis and quality of life, with a reduction in hospitalization and enhancement of long-term survival compared with what was reported in some early ICD clinical trials.[1,3,13,18,19] Despite this, the proportion of patients who experience SCD has not changed substantially. The absolute risk for SCD and overall mortality increases with worsening LV function; however, the proportion of deaths due to primary arrhythmic causes, compared with non-arrhythmic cardiac and noncardiac causes, changes with worsening pump failure and

functional impairment.[6,20] A higher proportion of SCD is observed in patients with mild to moderate symptoms of HF (New York Heart Association [NYHA] class II, III); these patients derive greater improvement in overall survival from ICD therapy than those with severe HF.[1,5,13]

Guideline Recommendations and Evidence for Efficacy of Primary Prevention Implantable Cardioverter-Defibrillator Therapy in Nonischemic Cardiomyopathy

The benefits of ICD therapy are most pronounced in the secondary prevention of SCD and overall mortality among high-risk patients with ventricular dysfunction who have already had a life-threatening arrhythmic event, making the probability of recurrence high.[1] For primary prevention, the indication for ICD implantation is in patients at enhanced risk for life-threatening ventricular tachyarrhythmias, mainly defined by the persistence of severe LV dysfunction and HF symptoms despite adequate medical therapy. Thus, current joint guidelines by the American Heart Association (AHA), American College of Cardiology (ACC), and Heart Rhythm Society recommend ICD therapy as a class I indication for patients with NICM, HF with NYHA class II or III symptoms, and a persistent LV ejection fraction (LVEF) of ≤35% despite GDMT (usually for 3 months), with meaningful survival of more than 1 year expected.[2,5] This contrasts with recent European Society of Cardiology (ESC) guidelines for HF, which changed ICD implantation for similar patients with NICM from a class I to class IIa recommendation.[3,4] Given these differences, it is important to evaluate the evidence from clinical trials and meta-analyses that led to the class I indication for ICD implantation in patients with NICM, as well as the more recent data (Danish Study to Assess the Efficacy of ICDs in Patients with Nonischemic Systolic Heart Failure on Mortality [DANISH] trial) that resulted in the recent changes to the ESC guidelines.[11,18] The DANISH trial took place in the era of improved medical therapy and use of CRT for HF, advancements that further improved survival and therefore affected the power of studies to show the efficacy of ICD therapy in these patients.

Primary Prevention Implantable Cardioverter-Defibrillators Randomized Controlled Trials in Patients with Nonischemic Cardiomyopathy

Five RCTs between 1997 and 2017 studied the benefits of ICD therapy for primary prevention in all types of patients with cardiomyopathy with severe LV dysfunction and HF with NYHA functional class I-III (**Table 1**). The Cardiomyopathy Trial

(CAT, 2002, n = 104)[7] and Amiodarone versus Implantable Cardioverter-defibrillator Trial (AMIO-VIRT, 2003, n = 103)[10] were terminated early due to futility. Mortality rates were lower than expected, resulting in underpowering. The Defibrillators in Nonischemic Cardiomyopathy Treatment Evaluation Trial (DEFINITE, 2004) enrolled 458 patients with NICM with an LVEF ≤36% and premature ventricular complexes or non-sustained ventricular arrhythmias.[9] ICD use plus GDMT failed to show a significant reduction in all-cause mortality compared with GDMT alone (hazard ratio [HR] 0.65, P = .08) despite a significant reduction in the risk of SCD with ICD therapy (HR 0.20, P = .006). The Sudden Cardiac Death in Heart Failure Trial (SCD-HeFT) included 2521 patients with an LVEF ≤35% due to ICM or NICM[8] and compared medical therapy with amiodarone, versus ICD therapy, versus placebo. The trial concluded that amiodarone had no favorable effect on survival, whereas ICD therapy reduced the overall mortality by 23% (HR 0.77, P = .007) with an absolute decrease in mortality of 7.2% over 5 years. SCD-HeFT was the only randomized trial to demonstrate a mortality benefit from ICD implantation in both ICM and NICM. A subsequent meta-analysis of the NICM groups from these four trials found an all-cause mortality reduction of 31% with ICD therapy (HR 0.69; P = .002). Based on these trials and meta-analysis, ICD implantation for the primary prevention of SCD in patients with NICM with an LVEF ≤35% was recommended as a Class I indication.[2]

More recently, the DANISH trial investigated ICD therapy versus routine GDMT in patients with symptomatic NICM with an LVEF ≤35% and N-terminal pro-B-type natriuretic peptide (pro-BNP) greater than 200 pg/mL.[11] This study showed that prophylactic ICD implantation successfully reduced SCD (HR 0.50, P = .005) but did not significantly impact all-cause mortality compared with standard GDMT alone (HR 0.87, P = .28). The DANISH trial differed from the SCD-HeFT and DEFINITE trials in several ways. There was significant utilization of CRT devices in the control and ICD groups (58% of patients), with 93% of patients who had left bundle branch block and QRS duration greater than 150 ms receiving CRT therapy. CRT therapy most likely resulted in lower-than-expected mortality due to improved cardiac function in both groups, possibly minimizing the benefit of ICD therapy. The use of GDMT was much higher compared with previous trials, which may have resulted in improved outcomes, and patients were older, resulting in a higher risk of dying from non-cardiac causes. The DANISH trial's inclusion criteria included

pro-BNP, raising the possibility of a larger number of patients dying from pump failure rather than from arrhythmic etiology.[16] The lack of benefit to overall survival or cardiovascular death rate observed during the median follow-up of 5.6 years in the initial study[10] persisted on an extended follow-up of 9.5 years.[18] Patients older than 70 years of age did not show a beneficial effect on all-cause or cardiovascular mortality, whereas those ≤70 years showed improvement in both. Sudden cardiovascular death was reduced in the overall population and in patients ≤70 years but not in those older than 70 years of age. These results have influenced physicians' decisions, especially in Europe, about the implantation of an ICD for the primary prevention of SCD in patients with NICM.[21] The results also prompted the Heart Failure Association of the ESC, in its updated guideline, to change the recommendation for primary prevention ICD to a lower level (Class IIa) in patients older than 70 years of age with nonischemic HF and reduced LVEF.[3,4] The updated 2022 American HF guidelines (AHA, ACC, and Heart Failure Society of America), however, keep the recommendation for primary prevention ICD implantation in both ICM and NICM with an LVEF ≤35% as a Class I indication.[5] The decision is supported by meta-analyses of studies of primary prevention ICD in NICM, including the DANISH trial, which still shows a survival benefit from ICD therapy, although with a weakened effect on survival.[16,22] Similar survival benefits have been observed in several registry-based observational studies and other meta-analyses.[14,15]

Meta-analyses

Since the DANISH trial, numerous meta-analyses have assessed the role of ICD therapy in patients with NICM. Golwala and colleagues[15] demonstrated that, despite the addition of the DANISH data, there was a 25% reduction in all-cause mortality with ICD therapy compared with GDMT alone (HR 0.77). Al-Khatib et al.,[14] in their meta-analysis that included 1874 unique patients (937 ICD, 937 medical therapy) from four randomized trials (CAT, DEFINITE, SCD-HeFT, DANISH), also showed a significant reduction in all-cause mortality with ICD use (HR 0.75; 95% confidence interval [CI], 0.61 to 0.93; P = .008). Another meta-analysis that looked at ICD therapy versus conventional care for primary prevention in ICM and NICM found an overall reduction in all-cause mortality (HR 0.81, 95% CI 0.72–0.91) and SCD (HR 0.44, 95% CI 0.17–1.12) with ICD therapy. A more recent meta-analysis looked at the mortality benefit of ICD therapy in patients with NICM stratified by

Table 1
Five randomized controlled trials of primary prevention ICD in patients with NICM

Trial	Year	Hypothesis	Total Patients	% NICM Patients	Inclusion Criteria	Overall Mortality	SCD
CAT[7]	2002	ICD vs OMT	104	100	LVEF <30% NYHA II–III	Terminated early due to futility	
AMIOVIRT[10]	2003	ICD vs amiodarone	103	100	LVEF <35% NYHA II–III NSVT	Terminated early due to futility	
DEFINITE[9]	2004	ICD vs OMT	458	100	LVEF <36% NYHA I–III NSVT or PVCs	No effect ICD 12.2% vs OMT 17.4% (HR 0.65; 95% CI 0.40–1.06; P = .08)	Reduced SCD ICD 1.3% vs OMT 6.1% (HR 0.20; 95% CI 0.06–0.71; P = .006)
SCD-HeFT[8]	2005	ICD vs amiodarone vs OMT	2521	47	LVEF <35% NYHA II–III	Reduced overall mortality ICD 21.4% vs OMT 27.9% (HR 0.73; 95% CI 0.50–1.07; P = .06	NA
DANISH[11]	2016	ICD vs OMT	1116	100	LVEF <35% NYHA II–III (IV if CRT) NT-proBNP >200 pg/mL	No effect ICD 21.6% vs OMT 23.4% (HR 0.87; 95% CI 0.68–1.12; P = .28)	Reduced SCD ICD 4.3% vs OMT 8.2% (HR 0.50; 95% CI 0.31–0.82; P = .005)

Abbreviations: CI, confidence interval; HR, hazard ratio; ICD, implantable cardioverter-defibrillator; LVEF, left ventricular ejection fraction; NICM, nonischemic cardiomyopathy; NSVT, nonsustained ventricular tachycardia; NYHA, New York Heart Association; OMT, optimal medical therapy; SCD, sudden cardiac death.

CRT use. In patients who received ICD therapy but were not eligible for CRT, there was a 24% reduction in mortality (HR 0.76; 95% CI 0.62–0.93; $P = .008$). In contrast, among patients with CRT, a CRT-defibrillator was not associated with reduced mortality (HR 0.74, 95% CI 0.47–1.16; $P = .19$) compared with a CRT pacemaker, suggesting that the stabilization of HF with CRT may also influence arrhythmic events and mortality.[23]

Contemporary Medications and Sudden Cardiac Death Risk

Improvement in medications and compliance with their use, as well as the introduction of novel therapies, have reduced overall mortality and the impact of ICD therapy in patients with HF. In the SCD-HeFT trial, 69% of patients were on a beta-blocker, 96% on an angiotensin-converting enzyme inhibitor or angiotensin receptor blocker (ACEi/ARB), and 20% on a mineralocorticoid receptor blocker, whereas in the DEFINITE trial, 85% were on a beta-blocker and 86% on an ACEi/ARB (mineralocorticoid receptor blockers not reported). In the DANISH trial, 92% of patients were on a beta-blocker, 96% on an ACEi/ARB, and 58% on a mineralocorticoid receptor blocker; 58% had CRT.

Novel HF medical therapies introduced more recently have further changed the medical landscape, with incremental beneficial effects on the long-term outcomes of patients with HF. Angiotensin receptor neprilysin inhibition (ARNI) improved survival in symptomatic patients with HF with reduced ejection fraction in the PARADIGM trial.[24] Subsequent analysis of the PARADIGM study on the effect of ARNI on SCD found that ARNI reduced SCD risk in patients who received an ICD (HR 0.49; 95% CI, 0.25–0.99) and in those who were eligible for but did not receive an ICD (HR 0.81; 95% CI 0.67–0.98). This effect was particularly evident in NICM ($P < .05$).[25] Furthermore, recent data show that sodium-glucose cotransporter-2 inhibitors and glucagon-like peptide-1 receptor agonists in patients with HF may further add to the reduction in overall and cardiovascular mortality, and therefore, the likely benefit of ICD for primary prevention may diminish as overall outcomes improve.[26]

Sudden Cardiac Death Risk Stratification in Patients with Nonischemic Dilated Cardiomyopathy

Currently, the severity of LV dysfunction and HF symptoms are the major determinants for selecting patients with NIDCM for primary prevention ICD implantation.[5] However, the sensitivity and specificity of these predictors for identifying patients who will

benefit from ICD implantation are not very high. Most patients who receive an ICD do not receive appropriate therapy for ventricular arrhythmia during the device's lifetime, and patients with an LVEF greater than 35% are at risk for SCD but do not qualify for ICD as per guideline recommendations.[27,28] Risk prediction for SCD in patients with NIDCM, therefore, remains challenging and involves the consideration of multiple factors, including the underlying substrate, the potential triggers, and other modulating factors. The challenge arises from the dynamic nature of the arrhythmogenic substrate that is not static at any time and also changes over time both at the structural and functional levels with progressive remodeling at the molecular (ion channel and regulatory pathways), metabolic (energetics and signaling pathways), functional (gene and protein expression), and structural (chamber dilatation and scarring) levels, contributing to progressive pump failure and enhanced arrhythmogenesis.[12,28,29] Moreover, the arrhythmogenic substrate that remains stable most of the time could be perturbed by dynamic influences, such as myocardial stretch, ventricular ectopy, ischemia, hypoxemia, alteration in electrolytes, neuromodulators or catecholamines with exercise, or other conditions of sympathovagal alteration or hemodynamic fluctuation. Several studies have explored the use of markers that characterize the arrhythmogenic substrate and triggers, including measures of autonomic dysfunction, abnormalities in myocardial depolarization and/or repolarization, assessment of electrical instability by noninvasive or invasive means, myocardial functional metrics, extent and patterns of myocardial scar, symptoms of hemodynamic instability, and genetic variants.[30–32] Although prognostically significant, the individual predictive value of these markers is low and not useful for clinical SCD risk stratification when used alone. Recent approaches for risk stratification based on scoring systems incorporating a combination of clinical, electrical, and imaging markers are promising and need further validation in patients with NIDCM.[33,34]

Identifying patients with nonischemic cardiomyopathy at high risk for sudden cardiac death who would benefit from implantable cardioverter-defibrillator implantation while receiving guideline-directed medical therapy

An individualized approach in risk stratification has been suggested to distinguish the high-risk individual who will benefit the most from an ICD implant from those in whom a more conservative approach is best suited, whether due to multiple comorbidities that increase the risk of non-sudden cardiac death or to the overall low risk of SCD in the current era.[20] It is becoming more difficult to show any further reduction in overall mortality with ICDs implanted for primary prevention in optimally treated patients with NICM.[35] Alternative risk markers to LVEF and functional class and new prognostic models that incorporate multiple risk parameters are needed to identify individuals who are at high-risk for SCD despite GDMT and would therefore derive additional benefit from primary prevention ICD implantation.[33–35] Emerging data on the presence and quantification of scar; scar morphology, location, and volume on myocardial imaging with gadolinium-enhanced magnetic resonance imaging (MRI); novel circulating protein and RNA-based biomarkers of myocardial injury, inflammation, and stretch; and high-risk genetic variants are likely to provide additional insight into risk prognostication.[30,31,36–42]

Risk stratification starts with a thorough evaluation to determine the etiology of NICM, age, presence of comorbidities, and the severity and extent of the underlying substrate. To assess SCD risk, it is important to define the etiology of the cardiomyopathy. NICM is considered to be depressed LV systolic function in the absence of significant coronary artery or valvular disease. In clinical practice, NICM is often regarded as secondary to post-viral illnesses, but a familial genetic cause can be identified in greater than 30% of patients with NICM.

Genetic Variants Associated with High Risk of Sudden Cardiac Death

It is important to identify genetic causes of HF and arrhythmogenesis since patients with genetic causes may present at an earlier age and have worse outcomes. Several studies have demonstrated a familial predisposition to SCD, most often with autosomal dominant inheritance.[17,43] Potential genetic variants associated with SCD risk have been identified, which can be useful for screening family members for a diagnosis at a preclinical stage, allowing earlier intervention.[41] Four genes that encode for lamin A/C (LMNA), titin (TTN), β-myosin heavy chain (MYH7), and cardiac troponin T (TNNT2) account for the majority of NICM cases. These variants are more likely to be detected in a first-degree relative of patients with NICM diagnosed at a younger age or with findings suspicious for a specific etiology such as early conduction disease at a young age, as seen with LMNA cardiomyopathy.[17] Titin mutations appear to be the most frequent genetic variants identified. Certain mutations caused by LMNA genes are particularly arrhythmogenic, are associated with a high risk of SCD in up to 46% of patients, and may manifest

with premature conduction disease, atrial and ventricular arrhythmias, increased SCD risk, and progression to end-stage HF at a younger age.[36,44] In LMNA mutation carriers, the presence of nonsustained ventricular tachycardia, an LVEF less than 45% at first evaluation, male sex, and non-missense mutations have been identified as independent risk factors for ventricular arrhythmia.[45] ICD implantation is recommended as a class IIa indication for the primary prevention of SCD in those with high-risk features (LVEF <50%, nonsustained ventricular tachycardia, atrioventricular delay, 5-year estimated risk ≥10%).[4]

Pathogenic variants in LMNA, PLN, RBM20, and FLNC genes are particularly associated with a greater risk of ventricular tachycardia and SCD.[36,41,46] Genetic risk scores utilizing combinations of high-risk genetic variants and clinical profiles may be useful to refine SCD risk prediction in the general population and in patients with heart diseases. Despite the promising emerging data, the role of genetic testing for SCD risk stratification is currently limited to select patients and families with suspected inherited arrhythmias and cardiomyopathies, such as NIDCM, arrhythmogenic right ventricular cardiomyopathy, and hypertrophic cardiomyopathy.

Besides genetics, inflammatory cardiomyopathy accounts for the majority of cases of NICM—up to 50% of cases in some studies.[47] Numerous viral infections have been linked to NICM. Previously, adenovirus and enterovirus were common. Presently, parvovirus and human herpes virus 6 are more prevalent.[48] In South America and Central America, Chagas disease is the most frequent infectious etiology characterized by NIDCM in the setting of protozoan Trypanosoma cruzi. Autoimmune diseases have been associated with NICM.[49–52] Cardiac-specific antibodies directed against cardiac myosin have been reported to be associated with NICM.[53] Detection of these antibodies is important as these disease processes may respond to immunosuppression. Sarcoidosis is another important entity that needs to be ruled out during the workup of NICM, as cardiac sarcoidosis accounts for 0.5% of cardiac transplantations in the United States, is associated with a high risk of malignant ventricular arrhythmias and conduction disease, and may require permanent pacemaker or primary prevention ICD implantation.[54,55]

Myocardial Scar Presence and Extent as Predictor of Ventricular Tachycardia in Nonischemic Cardiomyopathy

Myocardial scar, by creating heterogeneous conduction and unidirectional block, promotes electrical reentry and ventricular arrhythmia in patients with NICM and has been demonstrated to be a strong and independent marker of SCD risk.[56–58] Analysis of the area of interface between scar and surviving myocardium with late-gadolinium enhancement (LGE) on MRI provides a more direct pathophysiologic correlation to life-threatening ventricular tachyarrhythmias and risk of arrhythmic death.[57] In a prospective, longitudinal outcomes registry of 1020 consecutive patients with NICM who underwent clinical cardiac MRI for the assessment of LVEF and scar, the presence of scar and LVEF ≤35% were strongly associated with all-cause and cardiac death but only myocardial scar was significantly associated with SCD risk.[59] In another study of 339 patients with NIDCM and without severe LV dysfunction (LVEF ≥40%), significantly greater SCD or aborted SCD events were observed over a median of 4.6 years in those with mid myocardial wall LGE versus those without LGE (18% vs 2%) with an adjusted HR of 9.2 (after adjusting for age, NYHA class, and LVEF).[39] Cumulative data from many studies strongly support the role of cardiac MRI with LGE in the risk stratification of patients with NICM. In a meta-analysis of 29 studies in patients with NICM (n = 2948), LGE on cardiac MRI was significantly associated with the arrhythmic endpoint, which remained significant even among patients with non-severe LVEF (35%-43%).[60] Many investigators have therefore recommended that scar assessment by MRI with LGE as a marker for arrhythmogenic substrate and risk of SCD be included in selection criteria for primary prevention ICD placement.[40,56,59,61–63]

Age

Age at the time of NICM diagnosis is important to consider when assessing the impact of ICD implantation. In a prespecified subgroup analysis of the DANISH study, there was a significant interaction between age and treatment effect.[18] Patients ≤70 years of age were more likely to have a survival benefit from ICD therapy (HR for mortality 0.70; 95% CI 0.51–0.96; P = .03) compared with patients above the age cut-off (HR 1.05; 95% CI 0.68–1.62; P = .84).[62] Advancing age is associated with a higher mortality risk from non-sudden cardiac death causes that will not improve with ICD implantation.

Competing Causes of Death

Of the five RCT already discussed, only one (SCD-HeFT) was able to demonstrate a mortality benefit in a population that included both ischemic and nonischemic causes of HF. This is partly related to the higher risk of non-sudden cardiac death based on the patient's comorbidities. Guidelines recommend against ICD implantation in patients with advanced refractory HF (NYHA Class IV) or expectation of good-quality survival of less than 1 year.[2,4] The Seattle Heart Failure Model incorporates patient baseline characteristics, HF medications, and laboratory data to assess the prognosis and predict all-cause mortality in patients with HF. It has been shown to provide more accurate risk stratification for non-sudden cardiac death versus SCD in patients with ICM and NICM.[64,65]

Another risk score, the Seattle Proportional Risk Model (SPRM), measures the risk of SCD versus non-sudden cardiac death and incorporates characteristics that result in a higher relative likelihood of SCD.[66] These include younger age, male sex, low LVEF, NYHA functional Class II versus Class III/IV, higher body mass index, and use of digoxin. Conversely, comorbidities such as diabetes, hyper- or hypotension, renal dysfunction, and hyponatremia reduce relative SCD likelihood as estimated by SPRM. SPRM score was used to identify patients in the DANISH study population at risk of SCD who would benefit from ICD implantation.[34] In patients with SPRM scores above the median, ICD implantation was associated with reduced all-cause mortality (HR 0.63; 95% CI 0.43–0.94), whereas patients with an SPRM score below the median had no mortality benefit (HR 1.08; 95% CI 0.78–1.49, P for interaction 0.04). As healthcare providers stress the importance of shared decision-making with patients regarding ICD implantation, these risk scores provide additional data so that an individualized, informed decision can be made based on the risk of non-sudden cardiac death.

Electrocardiographic Characteristics

Markers of cardiac depolarization and repolarization abnormalities have also been studied to assess the risk of SCD in patients with NICM. QRS prolongation is an independent predictor of mortality in patients with HF.[67,68] Fragmented QRS (fQRS) noted on electrocardiography has been studied as a risk marker in patients with ICM and NICM.[69] In a meta-analysis that looked at patients with HF who had or were eligible for an ICD, fQRS was associated with a 1.5 times greater risk of ventricular arrhythmia. NICM patients with fQRS had a 2.6-fold increased risk of death compared with their ICM counterparts.[69]

Patients with the left bundle branch block and a QRS duration greater than 150 ms are considered eligible for CRT. The COMPANION trial evaluated medical therapy alone against CRT-pacemaker and CRT-defibrillator device in patients with advanced HF due to ICM and NICM and a QRS interval of at least 120 ms. CRT therapy was associated with a reduction in the composite risk of mortality and HF hospitalization.[70] With CRT-pacemaker, the secondary endpoint of overall mortality was reduced by 24%, whereas CRT-defibrillator was associated with a 36% reduction in overall mortality.

Echocardiographic Parameters

A decline in LVEF has been used as a marker of SCD in the decision to implant an ICD; however, LVEF alone has been shown to have poor sensitivity and specificity. A significant proportion of ICD implant patients never receive therapy and about two-thirds of patients with SCD have an ejection fraction greater than 35% at presentation based on one study.[71] Additional echocardiographic markers, including global longitudinal strain (GLS), have been associated with the identification of high-risk patients who would benefit from ICD implantation. GLS measures ventricular longitudinal shortening, which is prone to be affected in the setting of ischemic stress. To assess the relationship of echocardiographic markers with ventricular arrhythmias in NICM, GLS, and strain-derived mechanical dispersion were studied in patients with NICM and ICM.[72,73] Both parameters were independent predictors of arrhythmic events compared with LVEF (HR per 1% increase in strain 1.26, 95% CI 1.03–1.54; $P = .02$; HR per 10-ms increase in mechanical dispersion 1.20, 95% CI 1.03–1.40; $P = .02$).[72]

SUMMARY

As overall death and SCD rates in patients with NICM continue to decrease due to improvements in medical therapy and interventions,[23] it will be difficult to show a further reduction in overall mortality with ICDs implanted for primary prevention in optimally treated patients.[20] Alternative risk markers to LVEF and functional class are needed. New models for the risk stratification of SCD that incorporate multiple risk parameters, including clinical risk profile, echocardiography, and information such as MRI-based scar localization, patterns, and extent; circulating biomarkers; and genetic variants may be able to identify individuals with NICM on optimal GDMT at high-risk for SCD with severe and nonsevere LV dysfunction (LVEF >35%) who would derive additional benefit from primary prevention ICD implantation.[30,31,33,34,37,41,74,75] This will require incorporating these models into appropriately designed, large clinical trials to demonstrate additional benefits of primary prevention ICD compared with existing therapies for patients with NICM.

CLINICS CARE POINTS

- Although primary prevention implantable cardioverter-defibrillators (ICD) reduce the risk of sudden cardiac death in patients with nonischemic cardiomyopathy (NICM), data regarding the mortality benefit in patients with NICM, particularly the elderly and those with comorbidities and on guideline-directed medical therapy, is uncertain.

- A thorough evaluation of heart failure etiology, comorbid conditions, and electrocardiographic and echocardiographic data, as well as assessment of myocardial scar with cardiac MRI, is essential to identify high-risk patients who will benefit the most from ICD implantation.

- A sudden cardiac death risk assessment tool based on abovementioned characteristics that is validated in randomized trials is needed to help guide clinical decision making in this complex and heterogenous patient population.

FUNDING

None.

DISCLOSURES

None.

REFERENCES

1. Tsao CW, Aday AW, Almarzooq ZI, et al. Heart disease and stroke statistics-2023 update: a report from the American Heart Association. Circulation 2023. https://doi.org/10.1161/CIR.0000000000001123. Online ahead of print.

2. Al-Khatib SM, Stevenson WG, Ackerman MJ, et al. 2017 AHA/ACC/HRS guideline for management of patients with ventricular arrhythmias and the prevention of sudden cardiac death: a report of the American College of Cardiology/American heart association task force on clinical practice guidelines and the heart Rhythm society. Circulation 2018;138:e272–391.

3. McDonagh TA, Metra M, Adamo M, et al. 2021 ESC guidelines for the diagnosis and treatment of acute and chronic heart failure: developed by the task force for the diagnosis and treatment of acute and chronic heart failure of the European society of

Cardiology (ESC) with the special contribution of the heart failure association (HFA) of the ESC. Rev Esp Cardiol 2022;75:523.

4. Zeppenfeld K, Tfelt-Hansen J, de Riva M, et al. 2022 ESC guidelines for the management of patients with ventricular arrhythmias and the prevention of sudden cardiac death. Eur Heart J 2022;43:3997–4126.

5. Heidenreich PA, Bozkurt B, Aguilar D, et al. 2022 AHA/ACC/HFSA guideline for the management of heart failure: a report of the American College of Cardiology/American heart association joint committee on clinical practice guidelines. J Am Coll Cardiol 2022;79:e263–421.

6. Myerburg RJ. Sudden cardiac death: interface between pathophysiology and epidemiology. Card Electrophysiol Clin 2017;9:515–24.

7. Bansch D, Antz M, Boczor S, et al. Primary prevention of sudden cardiac death in idiopathic dilated cardiomyopathy: the Cardiomyopathy Trial (CAT). Circulation 2002;105:1453–8.

8. Bardy GH, Lee KL, Mark DB, et al. Amiodarone or an implantable cardioverter-defibrillator for congestive heart failure. N Engl J Med 2005;352:225–37.

9. Kadish A, Dyer A, Daubert JP, et al. Prophylactic defibrillator implantation in patients with nonischemic dilated cardiomyopathy. N Engl J Med 2004;350:2151–8.

10. Strickberger SA, Hummel JD, Bartlett TG, et al. Amiodarone versus implantable cardioverter-defibrillator:randomized trial in patients with nonischemic dilated cardiomyopathy and asymptomatic nonsustained ventricular tachycardia–AMIOVIRT. J Am Coll Cardiol 2003;41:1707–12.

11. Kober L, Thune JJ, Nielsen JC, et al. Defibrillator implantation in patients with nonischemic systolic heart failure. N Engl J Med 2016;375:1221–30.

12. Kadakia RS, Link MS, Dominic P, et al. Sudden cardiac death in nonischemic cardiomyopathy. Prog Cardiovasc Dis 2019;62:235–41.

13. Narins CR, Aktas MK, Chen AY, et al. Arrhythmic and mortality outcomes among ischemic versus nonischemic cardiomyopathy patients receiving primary ICD therapy. JACC Clin Electrophysiol 2022;8:1–11.

14. Al-Khatib SM, Fonarow GC, Joglar JA, et al. Primary prevention implantable cardioverter defibrillators in patients with nonischemic cardiomyopathy: a meta-analysis. JAMA Cardiol 2017;2:685–8.

15. Golwala H, Bajaj NS, Arora G, et al. Implantable cardioverter-defibrillator for nonischemic cardiomyopathy: an updated meta-analysis. Circulation 2017;135:201–3.

16. Beggs SAS, Jhund PS, Jackson CE, et al. Non-ischaemic cardiomyopathy, sudden death and implantable defibrillators: a review and meta-analysis. Heart 2018;104:144–50.

17. Pinto YM, Elliott PM, Arbustini E, et al. Proposal for a revised definition of dilated cardiomyopathy, hypokinetic non-dilated cardiomyopathy, and its implications for clinical practice: a position statement of the ESC working group on myocardial and pericardial diseases. Eur Heart J 2016;37:1850–8.

18. Yafasova A, Butt JH, Elming MB, et al. Long-term follow-up of Danish (the Danish study to assess the efficacy of ICDs in patients with nonischemic systolic heart failure on mortality). Circulation 2022;145:427–36.

19. Shen L, Jhund PS, Petrie MC, et al. Declining risk of sudden death in heart failure. N Engl J Med 2017; 377:41–51.

20. Myerburg RJ, Goldberger JJ. Sudden cardiac arrest risk assessment: population science and the individual risk mandate. JAMA Cardiol 2017;2:689–94.

21. Haugaa KH, Tilz R, Boveda S, et al. Implantable cardioverter defibrillator use for primary prevention in ischaemic and non-ischaemic heart disease-indications in the post-Danish trial era: results of the European Heart Rhythm Association survey. Europace 2017;19:660–4.

22. Kolodziejczak M, Andreotti F, Kowalewski M, et al. Implantable cardioverter-defibrillators for primary prevention in patients with ischemic or nonischemic cardiomyopathy: a systematic review and meta-analysis. Ann Intern Med 2017;167:103–11.

23. Theuns DA, Verstraelen TE, van der Lingen ACJ, et al. Implantable defibrillator therapy and mortality in patients with non-ischemic dilated cardiomyopathy: an updated meta-analysis and effect on Dutch clinical practice by the Task Force of the Dutch Society of Cardiology. Neth Heart J 2022. https://doi.org/10.1007/s12471-022-01718-3 (online only).

24. McMurray JJ, Packer M, Desai AS, et al. Angiotensin-neprilysin inhibition versus enalapril in heart failure. N Engl J Med 2014;371:993–1004.

25. Rohde LE, Chatterjee NA, Vaduganathan M, et al. Sacubitril/valsartan and sudden cardiac death according to implantable cardioverter-defibrillator use and heart failure cause: a PARADIGM-HF analysis. JACC Heart Fail 2020;8:844–55.

26. Kanie T, Mizuno A, Takaoka Y, et al. Dipeptidyl peptidase-4 inhibitors, glucagon-like peptide 1 receptor agonists and sodium-glucose co-transporter-2 inhibitors for people with cardiovascular disease: a network meta-analysis. Cochrane Database Syst Rev 2021;10:CD013650.

27. Sabbag A, Suleiman M, Laish-Farkash A, et al. Contemporary rates of appropriate shock therapy in patients who receive implantable device therapy in a real-world setting: from the Israeli ICD Registry. Heart Rhythm 2015;12:2426–33.

28. Goldberger JJ, Subacius H, Patel T, et al. Sudden cardiac death risk stratification in patients with nonischemic dilated cardiomyopathy. J Am Coll Cardiol 2014;63:1879–89.

29. Gutman SJ, Costello BT, Papapostolou S, et al. Reduction in mortality from implantable cardioverter-defibrillators in non-ischaemic cardiomyopathy

patients is dependent on the presence of left ventricular scar. Eur Heart J 2019;40:542–50.

30. Akhtar M, Elliott PM. Risk stratification for sudden cardiac death in non-ischaemic dilated cardiomyopathy. Curr Cardiol Rep 2019;21:155.

31. Arsenos P, Gatzoulis KA, Tsiachris D, et al. Arrhythmic risk stratification in ischemic, nonischemic and hypertrophic cardiomyopathy: a two-step multifactorial, electrophysiology study inclusive approach. World J Cardiol 2022;14:139–51.

32. Gatzoulis KA, Tsiachris D, Arsenos P, et al. Prognostic value of programmed ventricular stimulation for sudden death in selected high risk patients with structural heart disease and preserved systolic function. Int J Cardiol 2014;176:1449–51.

33. Hammersley DJ, Halliday BP. Sudden cardiac death prediction in nonischemic dilated cardiomyopathy: a multiparametric and dynamic approach. Curr Cardiol Rep 2020;22:85.

34. Kristensen SL, Levy WC, Shadman R, et al. Risk models for prediction of implantable cardioverter-defibrillator benefit: insights from the Danish Trial. JACC Heart Fail 2019;7:717–24.

35. Beggs SAS, Gardner RS, McMurray JJV. Who benefits from a defibrillator-balancing the risk of sudden versus non-sudden death. Curr Heart Fail Rep 2018;15:376–89.

36. Kayvanpour E, Sedaghat-Hamedani F, Amr A, et al. Genotype-phenotype associations in dilated cardiomyopathy: meta-analysis on more than 8000 individuals. Clin Res Cardiol 2017;106:127–39.

37. Dhindsa DS, Khambhati J, Sandesara PB, et al. Biomarkers to predict cardiovascular death. Card Electrophysiol Clin 2017;9:651–64.

38. Halliday BP, Cleland JGF, Goldberger JJ, et al. Personalizing risk stratification for sudden death in dilated cardiomyopathy: the past, present, and future. Circulation 2017;136:215–31.

39. Halliday BP, Gulati A, Ali A, et al. Association between midwall late gadolinium dnhancement and sudden cardiac death in patients with dilated cardiomyopathy and mild and moderate left ventricular systolic dysfunction. Circulation 2017;135:2106–15.

40. Muser D, Nucifora G, Muser D, et al. Prognostic value of nonischemic ringlike left ventricular scar in patients with apparently idiopathic nonsustained ventricular arrhythmias. Circulation 2021;143:1359–73.

41. Gigli M, Merlo M, Graw SL, et al. Genetic risk of arrhythmic phenotypes in patients with dilated cardiomyopathy. J Am Coll Cardiol 2019;74:1480–90.

42. van Berlo JH, de Voogt WG, van der Kooi AJ, et al. Meta-analysis of clinical characteristics of 299 carriers of LMNA gene mutations: do lamin A/C mutations portend a high risk of sudden death? J Mol Med 2005;83:79–83.

43. Asselbergs FW, Sammani A, Elliott P, et al. Differences between familial and sporadic dilated cardiomyopathy: ESC EORP Cardiomyopathy & Myocarditis registry. ESC Heart Fail 2021;8:95–105.

44. Wahbi K, Ben Yaou R, Gandjbakhch E, et al. Development and validation of a new risk prediction score for life-threatening ventricular tachyarrhythmias in laminopathies. Circulation 2019;140:293–302.

45. van Rijsingen IA, Arbustini E, Elliott PM, et al. Risk factors for malignant ventricular arrhythmias in lamin A/C mutation carriers: a European cohort study. J Am Coll Cardiol 2012;59:493–500.

46. van den Hoogenhof MMG, Beqqali A, Amin AS, et al. RBM20 mutations induce an arrhythmogenic dilated cardiomyopathy related to disturbed calcium handling. Circulation 2018;138:1330–42.

47. Kuhl U, Pauschinger M, Noutsias M, et al. High prevalence of viral genomes and multiple viral infections in the myocardium of adults with "idiopathic" left ventricular dysfunction. Circulation 2005;111:887–93.

48. Maisch B, Pankuweit S. Current treatment options in (peri)myocarditis and inflammatory cardiomyopathy. Herz 2012;37:644–56.

49. Caforio AL, Vinci A, Iliceto S. Anti-heart autoantibodies in familial dilated cardiomyopathy. Autoimmunity 2008;41:462–9.

50. Ryabkova VA, Shubik YV, Erman MV, et al. Lethal immunoglobulins: autoantibodies and sudden cardiac death. Autoimmun Rev 2019;18:415–25.

51. Xiao H, Wang M, Du Y, et al. Arrhythmogenic autoantibodies against calcium channel lead to sudden death in idiopathic dilated cardiomyopathy. Eur J Heart Fail 2011;13:264–70.

52. Li X, Sundquist J, Nymberg V, et al. Association of autoimmune diseases with cardiomyopathy: a nationwide follow-up study from Sweden. Eur Heart J Qual Care Clin Outcomes 2022;8:79–85.

53. Latif N, Baker CS, Dunn MJ, et al. Frequency and specificity of antiheart antibodies in patients with dilated cardiomyopathy detected using SDS-PAGE and western blotting. J Am Coll Cardiol 1993;22:1378–84.

54. Kazmirczak F, Chen KA, Adabag S, et al. Assessment of the 2017 AHA/ACC/HRS guideline recommendations for implantable cardioverter-defibrillator implantation in cardiac sarcoidosis. Circ Arrhythm Electrophysiol 2019;12:e007488.

55. Yafasova A, Fosbol EL, Schou M, et al. Long-term adverse cardiac outcomes in patients with sarcoidosis. J Am Coll Cardiol 2020;76:767–77.

56. Alba AC, Gaztanaga J, Foroutan F, et al. Prognostic value of late gadolinium enhancement for the prediction of cardiovascular outcomes in dilated cardiomyopathy: an international, multi-institutional study of the MINICOR group. Circ Cardiovasc Imaging 2020;13:e010105.

57. Balaban G, Halliday BP, Porter B, et al. Late-gadolinium enhancement interface area and electrophysiological simulations predict arrhythmic events in

patients with nonischemic dilated cardiomyopathy. JACC Clin Electrophysiol 2021;7:238–49.

58. Centurion OA, Alderete JF, Torales JM, et al. Myocardial fibrosis as a pathway of prediction of ventricular arrhythmias and sudden cardiac death in patients with nonischemic dilated cardiomyopathy. Crit Pathw Cardiol 2019;18:89–97.

59. Klem I, Klein M, Khan M, et al. Relationship of LVEF and myocardial scar to long-term mortality risk and mode of death in patients with nonischemic cardiomyopathy. Circulation 2021;143:1343–58.

60. Di Marco A, Anguera I, Schmitt M, et al. Late gadolinium enhancement and the risk for ventricular arrhythmias or sudden death in dilated cardiomyopathy: systematic review and meta-analysis. JACC Heart Fail 2017;5:28–38.

61. Di Marco A, Brown PF, Bradley J, et al. Improved risk stratification for ventricular arrhythmias and sudden death in patients with nonischemic dilated cardiomyopathy. J Am Coll Cardiol 2021;77:2890–905.

62. Elming MB, Nielsen JC, Haarbo J, et al. Age and outcomes of primary prevention implantable cardioverter-defibrillators in patients with nonischemic systolic heart failure. Circulation 2017;136:1772–80.

63. Masci PG, Doulaptsis C, Bertella E, et al. Incremental prognostic value of myocardial fibrosis in patients with nonischemic cardiomyopathy without congestive heart failure. Circ Heart Fail 2014;7:448–56.

64. Levy WC, Mozaffarian D, Linker DT, et al. The Seattle Heart Failure Model: prediction of survival in heart failure. Circulation 2006;113:1424–33.

65. Mozaffarian D, Anker SD, Anand I, et al. Prediction of mode of death in heart failure: the Seattle heart failure model. Circulation 2007;116:392–8.

66. Shadman R, Poole JE, Dardas TF, et al. A novel method to predict the proportional risk of sudden cardiac death in heart failure: derivation of the Seattle Proportional Risk Model. Heart Rhythm 2015;12:2069–77.

67. Kurl S, Makikallio TH, Rautaharju P, et al. Duration of QRS complex in resting electrocardiogram is a predictor of sudden cardiac death in men. Circulation 2012;125:2588–94.

68. Marume K, Noguchi T, Tateishi E, et al. Mortality and sudden cardiac death risk stratification using the noninvasive combination of wide QRS duration and late gadolinium enhancement in idiopathic dilated cardiomyopathy. Circ Arrhythm Electrophysiol 2018;11:e006233.

69. Engstrom N, Dobson G, Ng K, et al. Fragmented QRS is associated with ventricular arrhythmias in heart failure patients: a systematic review and meta-analysis. Ann Noninvasive Electrocardiol 2022;27:e12910.

70. Bristow MR, Saxon LA, Boehmer J, et al. Cardiac-resynchronization therapy with or without an implantable defibrillator in advanced chronic heart failure. N Engl J Med 2004;350:2140–50.

71. Stecker EC, Vickers C, Waltz J, et al. Population-based analysis of sudden cardiac death with and without left ventricular systolic dysfunction: two-year findings from the Oregon Sudden Unexpected Death Study. J Am Coll Cardiol 2006;47:1161–6.

72. Haugaa KH, Goebel B, Dahlslett T, et al. Risk assessment of ventricular arrhythmias in patients with nonischemic dilated cardiomyopathy by strain echocardiography. J Am Soc Echocardiogr 2012;25:667–73.

73. Melichova D, Nguyen TM, Salte IM, et al. Strain echocardiography improves prediction of arrhythmic events in ischemic and nonischemic dilated cardiomyopathy. Int J Cardiol 2021;342:56–62.

74. Li X, Fan X, Li S, et al. A novel risk stratification score for sudden cardiac death prediction in middle-aged, nonischemic dilated cardiomyopathy patients: the ESTIMATED score. Can J Cardiol 2020;36:1121–9.

75. Kayvanpour E, Sammani A, Sedaghat-Hamedani F, et al. A novel risk model for predicting potentially life-threatening arrhythmias in nonischemic dilated cardiomyopathy (DCM-SVA risk). Int J Cardiol 2021;339:75–82.

The War Against Heart Failure Hospitalizations
Remote Monitoring and the Case for Expanding Criteria

Ioannis Mastoris, MD[a], Kashvi Gupta, MD, MPH[b], Andrew J. Sauer, MD[b],*

KEYWORDS

- Remote patient monitoring • Pulmonary artery pressure monitoring
- Multiparameter remote monitoring • Remote monitoring indications

KEY POINTS

- Successful remote patient monitoring depends on constant interaction between patients and multidisciplinary clinical teams.
- Hemodynamic pulmonary artery pressure monitoring is effective in reducing heart failure hospitalizations.
- Multiparameter CIED-based monitoring has encouraging results and is more effective than single-parameter monitoring.
- Potential expanded indications for remote monitoring would include GDMT optimization; application to specific populations, such as LVAD patients; and subclinical detection of heart failure.
- Voice recognition and analysis, IVC diameter monitoring, and AI-based remote ECG are promising novel remote monitoring methods.

INTRODUCTION

The concept of remote patient monitoring (RPM), despite its tremendous growth in recent years, is not novel. Clinicians have used devices, such as weight scales and blood pressure cuffs, for a long time as adjuncts to remote management of heart failure (HF). These devices serve as tools for patient self-management. In RPM, abnormal values trigger communication with clinician teams resulting in medication changes (diuretics) and additional modification of guideline-directed medical therapy (GDMT) or antihypertensive therapy. However, it is not always appreciated that this is a simplistic type of remote device-assisted monitoring that has been widely used.

Bidirectional, frequent communication between patients and multidisciplinary clinical teams is requisite for effective and successful remote monitoring. The main principles of RPM are conceptualized in **Fig. 1**. As shown, there is a flow of clinical data through the monitoring modality toward the multidisciplinary clinical teams to interpret and assess clinical meaningfulness. Closed-loop communication between parties requires patient adherence to the remote monitoring modality and timely response from the clinical team. A successful outcome depends on appropriate and timely medical intervention, followed by close follow-up and repeated monitoring to assess the response and effectiveness of the intervention. Thus, any issue interfering with the remote

a Cardiology Division, Department of Medicine, Massachusetts General Hospital, 55 Fruit Street, Boston, MA 02114, USA; b Saint Luke's Mid America Heart Institute and University of Missouri-Kansas City, 4401 Wornall Road, Kansas City, MO 64111, USA
* Corresponding author.
E-mail address: asauer@saint-lukes.org

Cardiol Clin 41 (2023) 557–573
https://doi.org/10.1016/j.ccl.2023.06.001

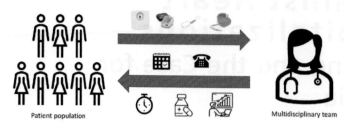

Fig. 1. Basic remote patient monitoring concept, a two-way street.

Patient population

Multidisciplinary team

monitoring feedback loop may render any strategy ineffective.

REMOTE EVALUATION OF VITAL SIGNS AND SYMPTOMS

Multiple studies have been conducted evaluating different strategies in RPM. TELE-HF, TIM-HF, BEAT-HF, and SUPPORT-HF2 are some of these studies that have deployed systems involving symptoms self-reporting through automatic voice messaging; "coaching" of patients with HF through regular telephone calls from dedicated HF nursing staff; predischarge HF education; provision of HF-related booklets for patient education at home; remote monitoring devices, such as portable weight scales, blood pressure cuffs, and electrocardiogram (ECG) devices; and regular follow-ups.[1–4] However, none of these trials showed effectiveness on the primary outcome, often a composite of all-cause mortality and HF hospitalizations, of the strategy in question **(Table 1)**. Ostensible explanations for not meeting their primary outcome include poorly selected patient populations (ie, low-risk populations), low patient adherence to the monitoring modality, inferior quality data, inadequate monitoring, or inadequate response to the data received from patients in the first place. Furthermore, setting a high bar with the primary outcome of all-cause mortality and readmission has rendered these trials with shorter follow-up times and modest sample sizes ineffective in detecting meaningful differences.

The Efficacy of Telemedical Interventional Management in Patients with Heart Failure (TIM-HF2) was a prospective randomized, controlled, parallel-group, unmasked trial of 1571 patients with New York Heart Association (NYHA) class II-III symptoms, HF with reduced ejection fraction (HFrEF; defined as ejection fraction [EF] ≤45%) or HF with preserved EF (defined as EF >45%) and concomitant use of oral diuretics, and recent admission to the hospital. The study adopted a structured monitoring intervention, including capturing changes in weight, heart rate, rhythm with ECGs, oxygen saturation, and self-reported patient health status.[5,6] These transmissions

occurred through the installation of an integrated telemonitoring system at the patient's home soon after randomization. An education curriculum on HF was provided initially and continued monthly through remote interviews with certified nursing personnel. In addition, patients were also equipped with a cell phone for calling in emergencies. Importantly, data received were processed by algorithms that allowed guided management and prioritization of high-risk patients. Through this detailed and intricate intervention, the study met its primary end point of reduction in the percentage of days lost because of unplanned cardiovascular hospital admissions or all-cause death in the RPM group (4.88%; 95% confidence interval [CI], 4.55–5.23) versus usual care (6.64%; 95% CI, 6.19–7.13; hazard ratio [HR], 0.80; 95% CI, 0.65–1.00; $P = .046$). The rate of all-cause death was 7.9 per 100 person-years in the RPM group and 11.3 per 100 person-years in the usual care group (HR, 0.70; 95% CI, 0.50–0.96; $P = 0.028$). There was no difference in the quality of life as assessed by the Minnesota Living with Heart Failure Questionnaire. Thus far, the TIM-HF2 trial has been the only study to date that a detailed monitoring strategy was found to meet its primary end point.

INVASIVE HEMODYNAMIC MONITORING: FACTS AND CURRENT CONCEPTS

Remote monitoring of vital signs and symptoms of HF has its inherent limitations. These do not pertain to the concept of remote monitoring per se. Instead, such regulations as quality and type of data collected, and timeliness of collection are more relevant. Even more critical is that symptoms of HF, such as worsening shortness of breath and weight gain, occur late in the trajectory of an acute exacerbation.[7] Chaundry and colleagues[8] showed that weight gain of greater than 2 lb occurs in 46% presenting with acute exacerbation, and whenever that happens, it precedes hospitalization by about 1 week. It has become more evident in studies of invasive monitoring that cardinal symptoms of HF and weight gain are poor predictors of future hospitalizations. Rising filling pressures precede clinical symptoms by a few weeks, indicating the

Table 1
Initial remote patient monitoring studies

Study	Year	Size	Key Selection Criteria	Intervention	Outcome	Potential Explanation for Success or Failure
WHARF[54]	1998–2000	280 (138)	• Adults 18 y and older • NYHA III or IV • LVEF ≤35%	• Follow-up: 6 mo • Parameters: Patient-reported symptoms and body weight • Other interventions: Response to monitoring: Responses reviewed by nurses and escalated to physicians based on the level of change in symptoms or weight	*Primary outcome:* 6-mo hospital readmission rate *Secondary outcome:* All-cause mortality, HF hospitalization, ER visitation, and quality of life	The trial did not show benefit likely because of the lack of involvement of physicians in the day-to-day monitoring of response to telemonitoring with delays in changes in medical therapy resulting in readmissions.
TEN-HMS[55]	2000–2002	426 (168)	• Adults 18 y and older • Recent admission for HF and LVEF <40%	• Follow-up: 240 d • Parameters: Blood pressure, heart rate, heart rhythm, and body weight • Other interventions: Response to monitoring: Values higher or lower than the threshold were reported to nurses who acted on the information or referred the query to the primary care physician	*Primary outcome:* Days lost because of death or hospitalization *Secondary outcome:* All-cause mortality, patient-reported symptoms, optimization of medications	The trial did not show benefit likely because of a stable patient population at recruitment.

(continued on next page)

Table 1
(continued)

Study	Year	Size	Key Selection Criteria	Intervention	Outcome	Potential Explanation for Success or Failure
Tele-HF[1]	2006–2009	1653 (826)	• Adults 18 y and older • HF hospitalization within 30 d based on HF admitting diagnosis, chest radiograph findings, and medication use	• Follow-up: 6 mo • Parameters: Patient-reported symptoms and body weight using a telephone-based interactive voice response system • Response to monitoring: Physician responded to answers submitted by patients and flagged for review on weekdays, not available on holiday weekends	*Primary outcome:* Any readmission or all-cause mortality within 180 d from enrollment *Secondary outcomes:* HF hospitalization, number of days in the hospital, and number of hospitalizations	The trial did not show benefit likely because of poor adherence to the intervention. Nearly 14% assigned to telemonitoring never used the device and toward the end of the study only 55% of patients were using the device at least 3 times a week.
TIM-HF[3]	2008–2010	710 (354)	• Adults 18 y and older • NYHA II or III • LVEF ≤35% and history of HF hospitalization within 24 mo or LVEF ≤25%	• Follow-up: Fixed stop date and median follow-up of 26 mo • Parameters: ECG, blood pressure, and body weight • Other interventions: Landline support in emergencies • Response to monitoring: Physician-led medical support 24 h a day 7 d a week with recommendations on medication titration, ambulatory assessment vs hospitalization	*Primary outcome:* All-cause mortality *Secondary outcome:* Cardiovascular mortality or HF hospitalization	Trial did not show benefit likely because of a stable patient population that was being optimally treated for HF. Furthermore, the analysis was limited by low statistical power to detect a difference in all-cause mortality.

Trial	Years	N (n)	Inclusion criteria	Monitoring details	Outcomes	Comments
BEAT-HF[2]	2011–2013	1437 (715)	• Adults 50 y and older • Hospitalized and receiving treatment of decompensated HF, with the expectation to be discharged to home	• Follow-up: 180 d • Parameters: Blood pressure, heart rate, body weight, and patient-reported symptoms • Other interventions: Predischarge HF education, scheduled telephone coaching • Response to monitoring: Nurse calls for abnormal values on parameters assessed with advice to follow with health care provider or present to emergency department	*Primary outcome:* All-cause readmission within 180 d after discharge *Secondary outcomes:* All-cause readmission within 30 d, all-cause mortality at 30 and 180 d, quality of life at 30 and 180 d	The trial did not show benefit likely because of poor adherence to the intervention. Also, the intervention was not integrated with the workflow of physicians providing care for the patients.
TIM-HF2[5]	2013–2017	1571 (796)	• Adults 18 y and older • NYHA II or III • Admitted within 12 mo for HF • LVEF ≤45% or LVEF >45% and on oral diuretics • Excluded patients with major depression	• Follow-up: At least 365 d • Parameters: ECG, blood pressure, and body weight • Other interventions: Mobile phone to contact telemedical center directly • Response to monitoring: Physician-led medical support 24 h a day 7 d a week with recommendations on medication titration, ambulatory assessment vs hospitalization	*Primary outcome:* Percentage days lost because of unplanned cardiovascular hospital admission or all-cause death *Secondary outcome:* All-cause and cardiovascular mortality	Trial was a success likely because of patient selection criteria and exclusion of patients with major depression, updated technologies with use of mobile phones, and convenience of transmitting information with the newer technologies.

Abbreviations: ER, emergency room; LVEF, left ventricular ejection fraction; NYHA, New York Heart Association.

latter are poor surrogates of the former.[7] Thus, invasive monitoring systems are uniquely placed in the early detection of augmenting pressures providing "lead" time for appropriate intervention and hospitalization prevention.[9]

The concept of impaired venous capacitance and increased stressed blood volume has received more attention in recent years with an evolving understanding of the pathophysiology of acute HF exacerbations. Under normal circumstances, the venous system contains approximately 70% of total blood volume because of its increased compliance compared with the arterial system.[10] Splanchnic veins are considerably more compliant than veins of the extremities. Highly vascular abdominal organs, such as the liver, spleen, and intestines, contain about 20% to 30% of the total blood volume representing a functional physiologic reservoir in the case of increased exercise or acute blood loss.[11] It is currently postulated that increased filling pressures occur because of impaired and decreased splanchnic venous blood capacitance mediated by the increased sympathetic tone that characterizes patients with HF.[12] That increase in sympathetic tone leads to the mobilization of fluid from the venous reservoir (unstressed blood volume) to the effective circulatory volume (stress blood volume), overwhelming the cardiac capacity to augment cardiac output in response to increased venous return without the elevation of filling pressures, thus culminating in the syndrome of congestion. Because of its nonlinear exponential relationship of venous blood volume with circulatory filling pressures, small changes in venous tone can achieve substantial changes in filling pressures.[13] The previously mentioned mechanisms would further explain the poor correlation of weight measurements in predicting future decompensations. Consequently, invasive hemodynamic monitoring may provide a more accurate way of averting HF readmissions and improving survival.

REMOTE PULMONARY ARTERY PRESSURE MONITORING

From the pivotal CardioMEMS Heart Sensor Allows Monitoring of Pressure to Improve Outcomes in NYHA Class III Heart Failure Patients (CHAMPION) study to the most recent Haemodynamic-GUIDEed management of Heart Failure (GUIDE-HF) trial, remote pulmonary artery (PA) pressure monitoring is a data-supported and reliable means of remote monitoring to reduce recurrent hospitalizations of patients with HF and recent history of acute decompensated HF

requiring inpatient admission for intravenous diuresis. The only Food and Drug Administration–approved monitoring system (CardioMEMS Heart Sensor, Abbott, Abbott Park, IL) consists of an implantable sensor, a delivery catheter, an electronic monitoring unit that contains a barometer to account for ambient atmospheric pressure changes, and a secure online database that facilitates transmission of individual patient clinical data to the responsible health care provider.[14] The sensor is implanted in a distal branch of the PA. Pressure changes in the PA are translated to changes to the circuit's resonant frequency. A summary of the clinical evidence supporting PA pressure remote monitoring is shown in **Table 2**.

CHAMPION was the first large-scale study to evaluate the safety and efficacy of PA pressure monitoring in 550 patients with recent HF hospitalization in NYHA class III HF. Six months after enrollment, there was an observed 28% (HR, 0.72; 95% CI, 0.6–0.85) reduction in HF-related hospitalizations in the treatment group. The observed effect was also sustained at 15 months of follow-up (HR, 0.63; 95% CI, 0.52–0.77).[15] A more aggressive GDMT uptitration was realized in the treatment group compared with the usual care group (9.1 vs 3.8 changes per patient; $P < .001$). An effect modification of GDMT through hemodynamic monitoring was suggested by Givertz and colleagues[16] in a secondary analysis of CHAMPION data. In patients receiving one element of GDMT along with hemodynamic monitoring, all-cause mortality decreased by 47% (HR, 0.63; 95% CI, 0.41–0.96), whereas those with two components (β-blockers, angiotensin-converting enzyme inhibitors [ACEIs], or angiotensin receptor blockers [ARBs]) had a more pronounced effect on all-cause mortality (HR, 0.43; 95% CI, 0.26–0.76).

The CardioMEMS Post-Approval Study (PAS) was a real-world, prospective, single-arm, observational study of 1200 patients with NYHA class III symptoms recruited from centers across the United States that underwent CardioMEMS implantation after an HF hospitalization within the past 12 months. Implantation dates spanned between September 1, 2014, and October 11, 2017.[17] Rates of HF hospitalization were compared between 1 year before and after implantation. Of those patients, 53% had low EF and had HFrEF, and 66.4% received a β-blocker and ACEi/ARB/angiotensin receptor / neprilyisin inhibitor (ARNI), whereas mineralocorticoid antagonists (MRA) were used in 54.6%. As seen in CHAMPION, medication changes were common among participants (an average of 1.6 medication changes per month), with 82.8% of patients receiving a medication change that would be

Table 2
Evidence supporting the use of remote pulmonary artery monitoring

Study	Size	Population Characteristics	Design (Follow-Up)	Outcomes	Results
Abraham et al.[14] 2011	17	NYHA III: Stable HF for 30 d before enrollment	Prospective, nonrandomized, single arm	Efficacy, accuracy, feasibility safety, intermediate-term safety	All implantation procedures without issues; 1 death noted that was not related to the procedure; correlation coefficients of 0.94, 0.85, and 0.95 for systolic, diastolic, and mean PA pressures agreement
CHAMPION[15] 2011	550	NYHA III for 3 mo; HF hospitalization within 12 mo	Prospective, randomized, multicenter, single-blind (hemodynamic monitoring vs conventional treatment; 6 mo)	*Efficacy:* Rate of HF hospitalizations at 6 mo postimplantation; delta in PA pressures; days alive outside hospital for HF-MLWHFQ *Safety:* device-related or system-related complications	Hospitalizations ↓ by 28% at 6 mo and by 37% in total follow-up; 98.6% freedom from complications; ↓ in PA pressures; days outside hospital ↓ by 6.7 d - MLWHFQ ↓ by 6 points
Heywood et al.[56] 2017	2000	All CardioMEMS implantations between June 2014 and September 2016	Retrospective, observational, single arm (6 mo)	*Efficacy:* delta in PA pressures compared with CHAMPION treatment arm at 1-, 3-, and 6 mo f/u Compliance with transmissions	Pressure ↓ by 32.8, 156.2 and 434.0 mm Hg* days at 1-, 3-, and 6 mo f/u, respectively; median of 1.27 d between transmissions after 6 mo
Abraham et al.[57] 2019	2174	Medicare beneficiaries with PA pressure sensor	Retrospective, matched cohort analysis (12 mo)	*Efficacy:* HF hospitalization, mortality, days lost because of HF hospitalization or death	HF hospitalization ↓ by 24%; mortality ↓ by 30%; days lost/pt ↓ by 28% because of death; days lost/pt ↓ by 27% for hospitalization or death

234

(continued on next page)

Table 2
(continued)

Study	Size	Population Characteristics	Design (Follow-Up)	Outcomes	Results
MEMS-HF 234.[58] 2020		NYHA III for 3 mo, HF hospitalization within 12 mo	Prospective, observational, multicenter, single arm (12 mo)	*Efficacy:* HF hospitalizations preimplant and postimplant - Delta in PA pressure preimplant and postimplant - KCCQ *Safety:* Freedom from device and procedure complications; survival	Freedom of complications 98.3%; survival 86.2%; hospitalizations ↓ by 62%; mean PA pressure ↓ by 5.1; KCCQ ↑ by 13.5 points
US Post-Approval Study.[17] 2020	1200	NYHA III: HF hospitalization within 12 mo	Prospective, open-label, observational, multicenter, single-arm (12 mo)	*Efficacy:* HF hospitalizations preimplant and postimplant; all-cause hospitalizations; transmission compliance; delta in PA pressures preimplant and postimplant *Safety:* freedom from device- or system-related complications, freedom from pressor sensor failure; survival	HF hospitalization ↓ by 57%; freedom from complications was 99.6%; freedom from sensor failure was 99.9%; all-cause hospitalization ↓ by 27%; survival at 1 y 83.9%; mean and median daily transmissions were 76% and 85%; PA pressures ↓ by 790 mm Hg* days
GUIDE-HF[18] 2021	1000	NYHA II-IV; HF hospitalization within 12 mo or BNP ≥250 pg/mL or NT-proBNP ≥1000 pg/mL	Multicenter, randomized, single-blind (12 mo); a prespecified pre-COVID analysis performed	*Efficacy:* Composite of all-cause mortality and total heart failure events at 12 mo; cumulative HF events; EQ-5D-5 L; KCCQ-12; 6MWT *Safety:* Freedom from device- or system-related complications	Overall all-cause mortality or HF event ⇔ pre-COVID all-cause mortality or HF event ↓ by 19%; overall cumulative HF events ⇔ pre-COVID cumulative HF events ↓ 24%; EQ-5D-5 L ↑; KCCQ-12 ↑; 6MWT ⇔

Abbreviations: 6MWT, 6-minute walk test; BNP, brain natriuretic peptide; EQ-5D-5L, EuroQol-5 Dimension-5 Level; f/u, follow-up; KCCQ, Kansas City Cardiomyopathy Questionnaire; NT-proBNP, N-terminal pro–brain natriuretic peptide.

considered GDMT optimization postimplantation. Total HF hospitalizations declined from 1600 before to 628 after implantation, with a risk reduction of 57% (HR, 0.43; 95% CI, 0.39–0.47; $P < .0001$). In 1-year survivors postimplantation, the rate of hospitalizations was also lower in the 1 year after implementation as compared with the 1 year preimplantation (HR, 0.35; 95% CI, 0.31–0.39; $P < .0001$). Survival at 1 year was 83.9% (95% CI, 81.7%–85.9%). A uniform risk reduction among different groups, irrespective of EF, was seen. Only five device- and system-related complications were reported (0.4%).

The recently published hemodynamic-GUIDEed management of Heart Failure (GUIDE-HF) trial expanded the knowledge base on remote monitoring in high-risk patients with HF.[18] GUIDE-HF assessed the composite of all-cause mortality and HF-related events in 1000 patients with NYHA class II-IV symptoms. Unlike CHAMPION, GUIDE-HF expanded the patient pool by including NYHA class II and IV and either elevated natriuretic peptides or recent hospitalization.[19,20] The primary outcome was a composite of all-cause mortality and HF hospitalizations or urgent HF hospital visits at 12 months. The COVID-19 pandemic impacted the results of GUIDE-HF. Overall, there were 253 events in the treatment group versus 289 events in the control group. No differences were found between the two groups for the primary and secondary end points during the study period. However, a prespecified pre-COVID-19 cohort analysis demonstrated benefit in the treatment group, irrespective of EF, on the primary outcome (HR, 0.81; 95% CI, 0.66–1.00; $P = .049$) that was primarily because of reductions in HF hospitalizations (HR, 0.72; 95% CI, 0.57–0.92; $P = .0007$). Subgroup analysis revealed noteworthy interactions for sex ($P_{interaction} = 0.01$) and race ($P_{interaction} = 0.095$), implying a more substantial treatment effect of remote PA pressure-guided management in women (HR, 0.64; 95% CI, 0.47–0.87) and Black patients (HR, 0.68; 95% CI, 0.48–0.97) compared with men and non-Black patients, respectively. No such finding has been previously demonstrated. It has been purported that such differences may represent a reduction in treatment bias (implicit bias) in addition to the fact that these two populations are disproportionately affected by HF and, thus, more likely to experience significant benefits with PA pressure-guided treatment. Finally, despite a higher degree of decrease in pulmonary pressures in the treatment group (area under the curve of −792.7 mm Hg-days [standard deviation, 1767.0] vs −582.9 mm Hg-days [standard deviation, 1698.1]) as compared with the control group, this did not translate to differential improvement in quality of life that was assessed using Kansas City Cardiomyopathy Questionnaire-12, EuroQol-5 Dimension-5 Level, and 6-minute-walk test. Because both groups experienced an increase in these scores, it has been suggested that this could be caused by unexpected improvement in the control group during the pandemic because of overall healthier patient choices during the emergency economic shutdown used by the US government in the first few months of the pandemic.[21,22]

In addition to PA pressure monitoring, the current PA pressure monitoring devices provide insights into ambulatory hemodynamics in various settings that allow individualized management of patients with HF. Frequent platform transmissions improve the understanding of ambulatory hemodynamics by providing measurements and visual waveform representation.[23] The latter can help understand unexplained exertional dyspnea (cardiac vs noncardiac); the longitudinal effect of GDMT uptitration; a waveform-based diagnosis of new-onset arrhythmias (eg, atrial fibrillation, supraventricular tachycardia) along with their impact on filling pressures; and impact of interventions, such as left ventricular assist device (LVAD) implantation and weight loss surgery (**Fig. 2**). In the setting of LVAD therapy, remote PA monitoring merits further consideration. Optimal hemodynamics during LVAD therapy have improved outcomes, led to medical optimization, and reduced LVAD-related complications.[24,25] Ongoing randomized studies, such as HEMO-VAD and INTELLECT 2, are currently exploring the impact of remote hemodynamic monitoring in patients with LVAD on future outcomes and quality of life.

CARDIAC IMPLANTABLE ELECTRONIC DEVICES

The increased prevalence of cardiac implantable electronic devices (CIEDs) in the cardiac populations, specifically in patients with HFrEF, has allowed for the development of newer technologies that facilitate RPM.[26] Sensors embedded within pacemakers and defibrillators provide an array of diagnostic information that may be useful to guide patient care remotely. These sensors can provide data on physiologic variables, such as heart rate variability, atrial and ventricular arrhythmia burden, thoracic impendence, the intensity of heart sounds, sleep incline, and physical activity.[27] Although single-parameter monitoring has provided initially promising results, their applicability in daily patient management has been limited by variable sensitivity/specificity ratios for

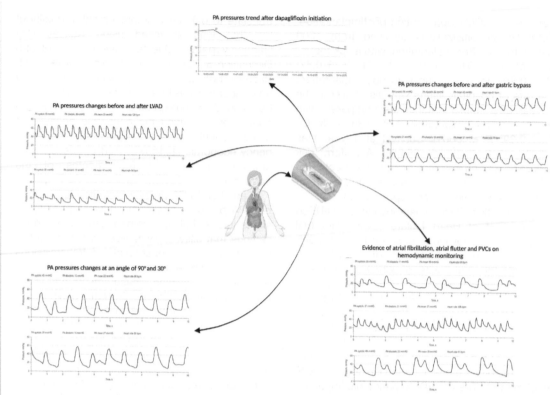

Fig. 2. Case scenarios of pulmonary artery pressure remote monitoring utility. (Created with BioRender.com.)

predicting HF-related events, depending on the set point of relevant thresholds.[28–30] Thus, integrating multiple physiologic parameters with concurrent hardware and software development is a natural evolution. Combining multiple parameters into a single metric prediction model has provided good discriminative power for future HF hospitalizations (**Table 3**).[31,32]

One such composite algorithm incorporates first (S1) and third (S3) heart sounds, thoracic impedance, respiratory rate, the ratio of respiratory rate to tidal volume (rapid shallow breathing index), heart rate, and patient activity to produce an index number using a proprietary algorithm. The index varies daily based on changes from the baseline based on variations in individual parameters. An alert requisite of further attention is produced when the index crosses a prespecified threshold.[33] The Multisensor Chronic Evaluation in Ambulatory Heart Failure Patients (MultiSENSE) trial evaluated the sensitivity of HeartLogic (Boston Scientific, Marlborough, MA) for HF events among intermediate- and high-risk patients.[34] Nine hundred patients were divided into derivation and validation cohorts and followed for 1 year while being monitored for prespecified HF-related end points. At a threshold of 16, the algorithm was deemed to exhibit the highest sensitivity (82%) with the lowest

unexplained alert rate (1.33/patient-year). The external algorithm validation yielded a sensitivity of 70% for HF-related events. The median lead time before an event was approximately 34 days, with 9 out of 10 patients having an alert onset at least 2 weeks before.

The Multiple cArdiac seNsors for mAnaGEment of Heart Failure (MANAGE-HF) trial provides a better framework in which remote monitoring offers an expanded platform besides hospitalization prevention. MANAGE-HF was a single-arm, observational, open-label study to evaluate the integration of HeartLogic in clinical practice and whether this would improve outcomes.[35] The study was designed in two stages, with phase I evaluating HeartLogic performance, changes in medical treatment, plasma natriuretic peptide levels, and HF hospitalization rates. In contrast, phase II will assess the efficacy of HeartLogic on future prediction of outcomes. Overall, 200 high-risk (prior hospitalization or increased natriuretic peptides) patients were enrolled and were prospectively followed for 12 months. The results of the first phase have been published. Notably, the study incorporated an alert management guide to ensure homogeneity in clinicians' responses, initially emphasizing decongestive therapies and GDMT uptitration while also addressing precipitating

Table 3
Multiparameter CIED-based remote monitoring studies

Study Name	Size	Population Characteristics	Design (Follow-Up)	End Points	Results
MultiSENSE[34] 2017	900	Boston Scientific CRT-D or ICD; NYHA II/III/IV	International, multicenter, nonrandomized	*End point 1:* Sensitivity to detect HFE >40% *End point 2:* Unexplained alert rate <2 alerts per patient-year	*Derivation group:* Sensitivity for HF detection was 82%, and the unexplained alert rate was 1.33 per patient-year *Validation group:* Sensitivity for HF detection was 70%; unexplained alert rate of 1.47 per patient-year; lead time before HFE of 34 d
MANAGE-HF[35] 2022	200	Boston Scientific CRT-D or ICD; LVEF ≤35%, NYHA II/III; hospitalization within 12 mo or unscheduled visit for HF within 90 d or BNP ≥150 pg/mL or NT-proBNP ≥600 pg/mL	International, multicenter, nonrandomized (21 mo)	Integration of HeartLogic in clinical practice, changes in medical treatment, changes in natriuretic peptides, changes in hospitalization rate	The HeartLogic alert rate at nominal threshold was 1.76 alert cases per patient-year HF treatment augmented in 74% of 585 alert cases NT-proBNP decreased from 1316 pg/mL to 743 pg/mL at 12 mo
SELENE HF[36] 2022	918	Biotronik CRT-D or ICD; LVEF ≤35%, NYHA II/III	Observational, international, multicenter, event-driven study	*Additional aim:* To develop a predictive algorithm, temporal trends of diurnal and nocturnal physiologic parameters by daily automatic RM were combined with a baseline risk-stratifier (Seattle HF Model) into one index *Primary end point:* First postimplant hospitalization for worsening HF *Secondary end point:* composite of any (first or subsequent) hospitalization, outpatient IVI, or death related to worsening HF	*Derivation group:* the index showed a C statistic of 0.89 with 2.73 odds ratio (CI, 1.98–3.78) for first HF hospitalization per unitary increase (P <.001) *Validation group:* sensitivity of predicting primary end point was 65.5% (CI, 45.7%–82.1%), median alerting time 42 d, and false (or unexplained) alert rate 0.69 (or 0.63) per patient-year

Abbreviations: BNP, brain natriuretic peptide; CRT, cardiac resynchronization therapy; HFE, heart failure event; ICD, internal cardioverter defibrillator; IVI, intravenous infusion; LVEF, left ventricular ejection fraction; NT-proBNP, N-terminal pro–brain natriuretic peptide; RM, remote monitoring.

factors for HF decompensation. During follow-up, there were 585 alert cases with an average of 1.76 alert cases per patient-year. HF treatment was modified in 74% of the participants with at least one alert. There was significant variation in the response by study sites regarding the medication classes; however, most changes involved diuretics, whereas GDMT optimization occurred less commonly. As expected, changes in medication regimen were more common when patients were in alert state (8.3-fold for all HF classes, 11.6-fold for loop diuretics, 24.7-fold for thiazide diuretics, 3-fold for ARNI/ACEI/ARBs, 2.6-fold for β-blockers, and 5.3-fold for vasodilators). The index decreased quicker when initial decongestive therapies were given. Finally, the HF hospitalization rate was 0.26 per patient-year, whereas the all-cause rate was 0.05 per patient-year. Heart-Logic was in alert status within 30 days preceding 83% of hospitalizations with HF as the primary reason for admission providing good discriminatory power.

On the same footprint that MultiSENSE was established, the Selection of potential predictors of worsening Heart Failure (SELENE-HF) study expanded knowledge based on CIED-based multiparameter monitoring.[36] SELENE-HF was an observational, multicenter, event-driven study that correlated remote monitoring data with clinical outcomes, including HF-related hospitalizations and deaths in 918 patients with internal cardioverter defibrillator or cardiac resynchronization therapy-D and NYHA class II or III. The study's design derived a new algorithm that integrated variables, such as heart rate variability, 24-hour activity, arrhythmia burden, and thoracic impendence. An innovative part of the algorithm was incorporating a risk-stratifying score, such as the Seattle HF model. They attempted to refine its predictive ability and prioritize patients requiring earlier medical intervention.[37] Although the study initially aimed at developing a prediction algorithm, the occurrence of more than expected events allowed for the derivation and validation of the intended algorithm. At a follow-up of 22.5 months, the derivation group consisted of 457 patients (31 end points) and the validation group of 461 patients (29 end points, respectively). In the derivation cohort, a unit increase of the index was associated with an odds ratio of 2.73 (95% CI, 1.98–3.78; $P < .001$) for the primary outcome with a respective receiver operating characteristic curve of 0.89 (CI, 0.83–0.95). At a nominal threshold of 3.5 and 4.5, the algorithm was associated with a projected sensitivity of 81.5% (95% CI, 61.9%–93.7%) to 63.0% (95% CI, 42.4%–80.6%) and a projected specificity of 82.6%

(95% CI, 78.2%–86.5%) to 90.7% (95% CI, 89.0%–94.9%), respectively. In the validation group, at a threshold of 4.5, the sensitivity was 65.5% with 42 days median alert time and a false alert rate of 0.69 alerts/patient/year. In contrast, a threshold of 3.5 performed slightly better with a sensitivity of 72.4%, albeit with a higher false rate (1.07 alerts/patient/year). A sensitivity analysis excluding the Seattle Heart Failure Model (SHFM) raised the false and unexplained alerts by 10% in both cohorts.

THE CASE FOR EXPANSION OF INDICATION CRITERIA

Over the past few decades, tremendous progress has been realized in RPM in patients with HF. Randomized clinical trials have studied various noninvasive strategies of vitals monitoring, invasive hemodynamic monitoring, and CIED-based multiparameter monitoring (**Fig. 3**). The early trials studied the composite outcome of HF-related hospitalizations and all-cause mortality in a stable high-risk outpatient HF population following a recent HF admission to the hospital. Although preventing further decompensation is paramount, optimizing their GDMT regimen and reducing their residual risk for disease progression is also crucial. Numerous studies have shown variable prescription rates of different GDMT classes and low rates of goal doses of GDMT because of delays in the uptitration of medications that can potentially reduce further mortality.[38] These observations are related to physician inertia, perceived side effects, risks associated with GDMT, and infrequent follow-up.[39] Rapid and timely uptitration of GDMT after initiation has provided incremental benefits in averting HF hospitalization and deaths.[40,41] In that context, refocusing remote monitoring studies outcomes toward assessing GDMT titration would be a plausible and reasonable next step. The current technology used by RPM devices provides a wealth of information, making remote titration of GDMT a tangible reality. The combination of remote monitoring platforms paired with remote creatinine and electrolyte monitoring would further boost this possibility.

In addition, remote hemodynamic monitoring may be of particular interest and add value in smaller specialized populations, such as those with mechanical circulatory support. Within the premises of this population, frequent hemodynamic assessment by catheterization has been associated with improved outcomes in addition to lower device-associated complication rates, such as right ventricular failure and device thrombosis that would further reduce rehospitalizations.

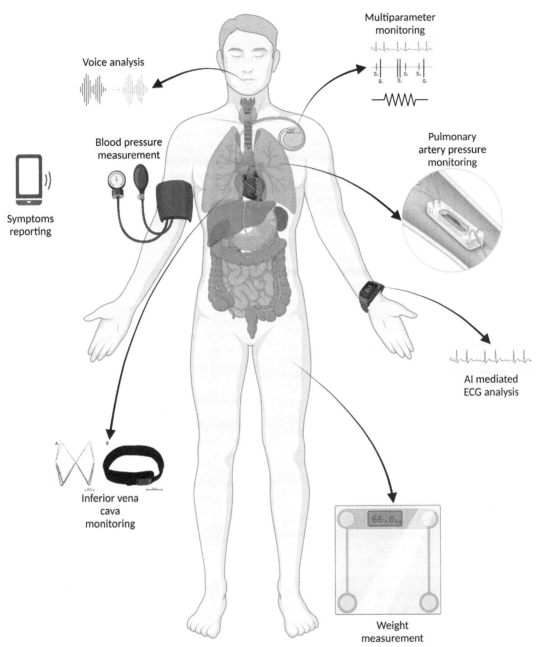

Fig. 3. Current and future target for remote patient monitoring in patients with heart failure. (Created with BioRender.com.)

Ongoing studies are also evaluating the feasibility of a closed-loop feedback controller that would result in transient speed adjustments based on elevated PA pressures.[42]

Finally, the development of artificial intelligence ECG-based monitoring through wearable devices provides a financially accessible and attractive way of monitoring large populations to detect arrhythmias in early asymptomatic HF (stage B). Although widespread monitoring of low-risk populations would neither be cost-effective nor appropriate, it is a reasonable strategy for patients at elevated risk as defined by the recent definition of HF (stage A).[43] The addition of remote N-terminal pro–brain natriuretic peptide assay testing would provide incremental benefits in these populations' early diagnosis and prognostication.[44,45] It is crucial to implement such strategies to create the framework for equitable and fair monitoring and treatment opportunities.

EMERGING TECHNOLOGY IN THE REMOTE MONITORING ARENA

With a further understanding of the pathophysiology underlying the mechanisms and the physiologic changes associated with HF decompensation, newer monitoring devices are being evaluated for their ability to avert HF hospitalizations and patient-perceived quality of life (see **Fig. 3**).

The importance of the splanchnic venous system in regulating stressed blood volume and the cardiac venous return has been described previously in this review. In this context, monitoring venous return through the inferior vena cava (IVC) is a plausible RPM target. Initial animal-based studies of resonance-based IVC sensors have provided promising results. The FIRE1 sensor is a chronic implantable passive monitor to measure the cross-sectional area of the IVC over time.[46] The sensor was implanted between renal and hepatic veins in nine sheep via femoral access. The sensor was initially validated ex vivo and in vivo and then used to correlate the cross-sectional area of the IVC during three distinct experiments (volume infusion, vasodilation via nitro infusion, and cardiac dysfunction through rapid pacing) with right-sided filling pressures. IVC area changes were more sensitive than changes in cardiac filling pressures during colloid infusion ($P < .001$), vasodilatation ($P < .001$), and cardiac dysfunction induced by rapid pacing ($P \leq .02$). The mean time from detection in the IVC area changes until significant changes in filling pressure is not provided. Whether these earlier changes are clinically meaningful warrants further investigation.

Artificial intelligence–based electrocardiography has been evaluated as a screening modality for the early detection of subclinical LV dysfunction. Although low EF does not readily translate into symptomatic HF, early detection has important prognostic and therapeutic ramifications.[47] Several studies have evaluated the potential of different artificial intelligence ECG algorithms in detecting subclinical LV dysfunction. These models have deployed deep learning convolutional neural networks to associate ECG with echocardiographic data and have trained them to diagnose LV dysfunction on an ECG alone. These models have exhibited impressive performance with sensitivity, and specificity greater than 85% and area under the curve of approximately 0.91 to 0.93.[48,49] The remote identification of atrial fibrillation through a single-lead ECG via a smartwatch was recently demonstrated.[50] A recent study also showed that a smartwatch-enabled ECG-based algorithm detected LV dysfunction with an area under the curve ranging from 0.885 (95% CI,

0.823–0.946) to 0.881 (95% CI, 0.815–0.947). Further studies are warranted to discern the predictive accuracy of ECG-based algorithms in the detection of HFrEF.[51]

The value of speech analysis via a speech processing algorithm for evaluating patients with HF has been explored. It has been purported that in a HF state, altered phonation patterns may be able to detect fluid overload and pulmonary congestion. Maor and colleagues[52] have shown that a vocal biomarker derived from a recorded patient message was associated with increased death and hospitalization risk with increasing patient quartiles of the biomarker. The feasibility of detecting voice alterations indicative of HF status was confirmed by a different study in which 40 patients were recorded through a remote proprietary speech analysis application tool.[53] More specifically, the application could identify differences in five distinct voice measures between "congested" and "dry" conditions on admission and discharge because of HF decompensation. Thus, remote voice mechanics analysis may provide a valuable tool in the armamentarium of available HF hospitalization reduction modalities.

SUMMARY

The available remote monitoring platforms have grown exponentially in recent significant technological advancements. Many physiologic parameters can be monitored using noninvasive and invasive strategies. The battery of available platforms gives the HF community unprecedented power to avert adverse outcomes and improve provided care in a timely fashion. To harness that power, further implementation studies are required to assess the feasibility and effectiveness of remote care delivery regarding GDMT optimization.

CLINICS CARE POINTS

- Remote monitoring has a long history of development and most studies of home telemonitoring have failed to demonstrate major impact on reducing patient morbidity or mortality.

- Invasive remote pulmonary artery pressure monitoring has been shown to reduce hospitalizations for heart failure in pivotal clinical trials and in real-world observational studies, with promise for assisting safe and more aggressive initiation and titration of guideline-directed medical therapies.

- Future innovation in digital health technologies involved in remote patient monitoring may incorporate measurements of unstressed blood volume, voice change technology, multivariable heart rate and heart rhythm algorithms incorporating artificial intelligence, and other technologies incorporating bioimpedence, seismocardiography, and acoustic monitoring.

DISCLOSURE

Dr A.J. Sauer reports receiving compensation from Abbott, Boston Scientific, Biotronik, Acorai, Story Health, General Prognostics, and Impulse Dynamics for advising, speaking, and performing research activities. Dr I. Mastoris has no relevant disclosures to this work. Dr K. Gupta has no relevant disclosures to this work.

REFERENCES

1. Chaudhry SI, Mattera JA, Curtis JP, et al. Telemonitoring in patients with heart failure. N Engl J Med 2010;363(24):2301–9. https://doi.org/10.1056/nejmoa1010029.

2. Ong MK, Romano PS, Edgington S, et al. Effectiveness of remote patient monitoring after discharge of hospitalized patients with heart failure. JAMA Intern Med 2016;176(3):310. https://doi.org/10.1001/jamainternmed.2015.7712.

3. Koehler F, Winkler S, Schieber M, et al. Impact of remote telemedical management on mortality and hospitalizations in ambulatory patients with chronic heart failure: the telemedical interventional monitoring in heart failure study. Circulation 2011;123(17):1873–80. https://doi.org/10.1161/circulationaha.111.018473.

4. Rahimi K, Nazarzadeh M, Pinho-Gomes A-C, et al. Home monitoring with technology-supported management in chronic heart failure: a randomised trial. Heart 2020;106(20):1573–8. https://doi.org/10.1136/heartjnl-2020-316773.

5. Koehler F, Koehler K, Deckwart O, et al. Efficacy of telemedical interventional management in patients with heart failure (TIM-HF2): a randomised, controlled, parallel-group, unmasked trial. Lancet 2018;392(10152):1047–57. https://doi.org/10.1016/s0140-6736(18)31880-4.

6. Koehler F, Koehler K, Deckwart O, et al. Telemedical Interventional Management in Heart Failure II (TIM-HF2), a randomised, controlled trial investigating the impact of telemedicine on unplanned cardiovascular hospitalisations and mortality in heart failure patients: study design and description. Eur J Heart Fail 2018;20(10):1485–93. https://doi.org/10.1002/ejhf.1300.

7. Zile MR, Bennett TD, John Sutton M, et al. Transition from chronic compensated to acute decompensated heart failure. Circulation 2008;118(14):1433–41. https://doi.org/10.1161/circulationaha.108.783910.

8. Chaudhry SI, Wang Y, Concato J, et al. Patterns of weight change preceding hospitalization for heart failure. Circulation 2007;116(14):1549–54. https://doi.org/10.1161/circulationaha.107.690768.

9. Abraham WT, Perl L. Implantable hemodynamic monitoring for heart failure patients. J Am Coll Cardiol 2017;70(3):389–98. https://doi.org/10.1016/j.jacc.2017.05.052.

10. Gelman S. Venous function and central venous pressure: a physiologic story. Anesthesiology 2008;108(4):735–48. https://doi.org/10.1097/ALN.0b013e3181672607.

11. Fudim M, Kaye DM, Borlaug BA, et al. Venous tone and stressed blood volume in heart failure: JACC review topic of the week. J Am Coll Cardiol 2022;79(18):1858–69. https://doi.org/10.1016/j.jacc.2022.02.050.

12. Fallick C, Sobotka PA, Dunlap ME. Sympathetically mediated changes in capacitance. Circulation: Heart Fail 2011;4(5):669–75. https://doi.org/10.1161/circheartfailure.111.961789.

13. Rothe CF. Physiology of venous return: an unappreciated boost to the heart. Arch Intern Med 1986;146(5):977–82. https://doi.org/10.1001/archinte.1986.00360170223028.

14. Abraham WT, Adamson PB, Hasan A, et al. Safety and accuracy of a wireless pulmonary artery pressure monitoring system in patients with heart failure. Am Heart J 2011;161(3):558–66. https://doi.org/10.1016/j.ahj.2010.10.041.

15. Abraham WT, Adamson PB, Bourge RC, et al. Wireless pulmonary artery haemodynamic monitoring in chronic heart failure: a randomised controlled trial. Lancet 2011;377(9766):658–66. https://doi.org/10.1016/s0140-6736(11)60101-3.

16. Givertz MM, Stevenson LW, Costanzo MR, et al. Pulmonary artery pressure-guided management of patients with heart failure and reduced ejection fraction. J Am Coll Cardiol 2017;70(15):1875–86. https://doi.org/10.1016/j.jacc.2017.08.010.

17. Shavelle DM, Desai AS, Abraham WT, et al. Lower rates of heart failure and all-cause hospitalizations during pulmonary artery pressure-guided therapy for ambulatory heart failure. Circulation: Heart Fail 2020;13(8). https://doi.org/10.1161/circheartfailure.119.006863.

18. Lindenfeld J, Zile MR, Desai AS, et al. Haemodynamic-guided management of heart failure (GUIDE-HF): a randomised controlled trial. Lancet 2021;398(10304):991–1001. https://doi.org/10.1016/s0140-6736(21)01754-2.

19. Januzzi JL, Zannad F, Anker SD, et al. Prognostic importance of NT-proBNP and effect of

empagliflozin in the EMPEROR-reduced trial. J Am Coll Cardiol 2021;78(13):1321–32. https://doi.org/10.1016/j.jacc.2021.07.046.

20. Zile MR, Claggett BL, Prescott MF, et al. Prognostic implications of changes in N-terminal pro-B-type natriuretic peptide in patients with heart failure. J Am Coll Cardiol 2016/12/06/2016;68(22):2425–36.

21. O'Connell M, Smith K, Stroud R. The dietary impact of the COVID-19 pandemic. J Health Econ 2022/07/01/2022;84:102641.

22. Bennett G, Young E, Butler I, et al. The impact of lockdown during the COVID-19 outbreak on dietary habits in various population groups: a scoping review. Review. Frontiers in Nutrition 2021;8. https://doi.org/10.3389/fnut.2021.626432. doi:.

23. Alam A, Jermyn R, Mastoris I, et al. Ambulatory factors influencing pulmonary artery pressure waveforms and implications for clinical practice. Heart Fail Rev 2022. https://doi.org/10.1007/s10741-022-10249-3.

24. Imamura T, Nguyen A, Kim G, et al. Optimal haemodynamics during left ventricular assist device support are associated with reduced haemocompatibility: related adverse events. Eur J Heart Fail 2019;21(5):655–62. https://doi.org/10.1002/ejhf.1372.

25. Imamura T, Jeevanandam V, Kim G, et al. Optimal hemodynamics during left ventricular assist device support are associated with reduced readmission rates. Circulation: Heart Fail 2019;12(2). https://doi.org/10.1161/circheartfailure.118.005094.

26. Voigt A, Shalaby A, Saba S. Continued rise in rates of cardiovascular implantable electronic device infections in the United States: temporal trends and causative insights. Pacing Clin Electrophysiol 2010;33(4):414–9. https://doi.org/10.1111/j.1540-8159.2009.02569.x.

27. Mastoris I, Spall HGCV, Sheldon SH, et al. Emerging implantable-device technology for patients at the intersection of electrophysiology and heart failure interdisciplinary care. J Card Fail 2021. https://doi.org/10.1016/j.cardfail.2021.11.006.

28. Domenichini G, Rahneva T, Diab IG, et al. The lung impedance monitoring in treatment of chronic heart failure (the LIMIT-CHF study). Europace 2016;18(3):428–35. https://doi.org/10.1093/europace/euv293.

29. Van Veldhuisen DJ, Braunschweig F, Conraads V, et al. Intrathoracic impedance monitoring, audible patient alerts, and outcome in patients with heart failure. Circulation 2011;124(16):1719–26. https://doi.org/10.1161/circulationaha.111.043042.

30. Vollmann D, Nägele H, Schauerte P, et al. Clinical utility of intrathoracic impedance monitoring to alert patients with an implanted device of deteriorating chronic heart failure. Eur Heart J 2007;28(15):1835–40. https://doi.org/10.1093/eurheartj/ehl506.

31. Cowie MR, Sarkar S, Koehler J, et al. Development and validation of an integrated diagnostic algorithm derived from parameters monitored in implantable devices for identifying patients at risk for heart failure hospitalization in an ambulatory setting. Eur Heart J 2013;34(31):2472–80. https://doi.org/10.1093/eurheartj/eht083.

32. Virani SA, Sharma V, McCann M, et al. Prospective evaluation of integrated device diagnostics for heart failure management: results of the TRIAGE-HF study. ESC Heart Fail 2018;5(5):809–17. https://doi.org/10.1002/ehf2.12309.

33. Siejko KZ, Thakur PH, Maile K, et al. Feasibility of heart sounds measurements from an accelerometer within an ICD pulse generator. Pacing Clin Electrophysiol 2013;36(3):334–46. https://doi.org/10.1111/pace.12059.

34. Boehmer JP, Hariharan R, Devecchi FG, et al. A multisensor algorithm predicts heart failure events in patients with implanted devices. JACC (J Am Coll Cardiol): Heart Fail 2017;5(3):216–25. https://doi.org/10.1016/j.jchf.2016.12.011.

35. Hernandez AF, Albert NM, Allen LA, et al. Multiple cArdiac seNsors for mAnaGEment of heart failure (MANAGE-HF): phase I evaluation of the integration and safety of the HeartLogic multisensor algorithm in patients with heart failure. J Card Fail 2022;28(8):1245–54. https://doi.org/10.1016/j.cardfail.2022.03.349.

36. D'Onofrio A, Solimene F, Calò L, et al. Combining home monitoring temporal trends from implanted defibrillators and baseline patient risk profile to predict heart failure hospitalizations: results from the SELENE HF study. EP Europace 2022;24(2):234–44. https://doi.org/10.1093/europace/euab170.

37. Levy WC, Mozaffarian D, Linker DT, et al. The Seattle heart failure model. Circulation 2006;113(11):1424–33. https://doi.org/10.1161/circulationaha.105.584102.

38. Greene SJ, Butler J, Albert NM, et al. Medical therapy for heart failure with reduced ejection fraction. J Am Coll Cardiol 2018;72(4):351–66. https://doi.org/10.1016/j.jacc.2018.04.070.

39. Savarese G, Kishi T, Vardeny O, et al. Heart failure drug treatment: inertia, titration, and discontinuation. JACC (J Am Coll Cardiol): Heart Fail 2023;11(1):1–14. https://doi.org/10.1016/j.jchf.2022.08.009.

40. Shen L, Jhund PS, Docherty KF, et al. Accelerated and personalized therapy for heart failure with reduced ejection fraction. Eur Heart J 2022;43(27):2573–87. https://doi.org/10.1093/eurheartj/ehac210.

41. Mebazaa A, Davison B, Chioncel O, et al. Safety, tolerability and efficacy of up-titration of guideline-directed medical therapies for acute heart failure (STRONG-HF): a multinational, open-label, randomised, trial. Lancet 2022/12/03/2022;400(10367):1938–52.

42. Veenis JF, Brugts JJ. Remote monitoring for better management of LVAD patients: the potential benefits of CardioMEMS. General Thoracic and Cardiovascular Surgery 2020/03/01 2020;68(3):209–18. https://doi.org/10.1007/s11748-020-01286-6.

43. Bozkurt B, Coats AJ, Tsutsui H, et al. Universal definition and classification of heart failure. J Card Fail 2021;27(4):387–413. https://doi.org/10.1016/j.cardfail.2021.01.022.

44. Mueller C, McDonald K, De Boer RA, et al. Heart Failure Association of the European Society of Cardiology practical guidance on the use of natriuretic peptide concentrations. Eur J Heart Fail 2019; 21(6):715–31. https://doi.org/10.1002/ejhf.1494.

45. Vergaro G, Gentile F, Meems LMG, et al. NT-proBNP for risk prediction in heart failure. JACC (J Am Coll Cardiol): Heart Fail 2021;9(9):653–63. https://doi.org/10.1016/j.jchf.2021.05.014.

46. Ivey-Miranda JB, Wetterling F, Gaul R, et al. Changes in inferior vena cava area represent a more sensitive metric than changes in filling pressures during experimental manipulation of intravascular volume and tone. Eur J Heart Fail 2022;24(3): 455–62. https://doi.org/10.1002/ejhf.2395.

47. Wang TJ, Evans JC, Benjamin EJ, et al. Natural history of asymptomatic left ventricular systolic dysfunction in the community. Circulation 2003; 108(8):977–82. https://doi.org/10.1161/01.cir.0000085166.44904.79.

48. Siontis KC, Noseworthy PA, Attia ZI, et al. Artificial intelligence-enhanced electrocardiography in cardiovascular disease management. Nat Rev Cardiol 2021;18(7):465–78. https://doi.org/10.1038/s41569-020-00503-2.

49. Yao X, Rushlow DR, Inselman JW, et al. Artificial intelligence–enabled electrocardiograms to identify patients with low ejection fraction: a pragmatic, randomized clinical trial. Nat Med 2021/05/01 2021; 27(5):815–9. https://doi.org/10.1038/s41591-021-01335-4.

50. Perez MV, Mahaffey KW, Hedlin H, et al. Large-scale assessment of a smartwatch to identify atrial fibrillation. N Engl J Med 2019;381(20):1909–17. https://doi.org/10.1056/nejmoa1901183.

51. Attia ZI, Harmon DM, Dugan J, et al. Prospective evaluation of smartwatch-enabled detection of left ventricular dysfunction. Nat Med 2022/12/01 2022; 28(12):2497–503. https://doi.org/10.1038/s41591-022-02053-1.

52. Maor E, Perry D, Mevorach D, et al. Vocal biomarker is associated with hospitalization and mortality among heart failure patients. J Am Heart Assoc 2020;9(7). https://doi.org/10.1161/jaha.119.013359.

53. Amir O, Abraham WT, Azzam ZS, et al. Remote speech analysis in the evaluation of hospitalized patients with acute decompensated heart failure. JACC (J Am Coll Cardiol): Heart Fail 2022;10(1): 41–9. https://doi.org/10.1016/j.jchf.2021.08.008.

54. Goldberg LR, Piette JD, Walsh MN, et al. Randomized trial of a daily electronic home monitoring system in patients with advanced heart failure: the Weight Monitoring in Heart Failure (WHARF) trial. Am Heart J 2003;146(4):705–12. https://doi.org/10.1016/s0002-8703(03)00393-4.

55. Cleland JG, Louis AA, Rigby AS, et al. Noninvasive home telemonitoring for patients with heart failure at high risk of recurrent admission and death: the Trans-European Network-Home-Care Management System (TEN-HMS) study. J Am Coll Cardiol 2005; 45(10):1654–64. https://doi.org/10.1016/j.jacc.2005.01.050.

56. Heywood JT, Jermyn R, Shavelle D, et al. Impact of practice-based management of pulmonary artery pressures in 2000 patients implanted with the CardioMEMS sensor. Circulation 2017;135(16):1509–17. https://doi.org/10.1161/circulationaha.116.026184.

57. Abraham J, Bharmi R, Jonsson O, et al. Association of ambulatory hemodynamic monitoring of heart failure with clinical outcomes in a concurrent matched cohort analysis. JAMA Cardiology 2019;4(6):556. https://doi.org/10.1001/jamacardio.2019.1384.

58. Angermann CE, Assmus B, Anker SD, et al. Pulmonary artery pressure-guided therapy in ambulatory patients with symptomatic heart failure: the CardioMEMS European Monitoring Study for Heart. Eur J Heart Fail 2020;22(10):1891–901. https://doi.org/10.1002/ejhf.1943.

Secondary Mitral Regurgitation and Transcatheter Mitral Valve Therapies
Do They Have a Role in Advanced Heart Failure with Reduced Ejection Fraction?

Michael J. Pienta, MD, MS*, Matthew A. Romano, MD

KEYWORDS

- Transcatheter mitral valve repair • Transcatheter edge-to-edge repair
- Secondary mitral regurgitation • Heart failure

KEY POINTS

- The Cardiovascular Outcomes Assessment of the MitraClip Percutaneous Therapy and Percutaneous Repair with MitraClip for Severe Functional/Secondary Mitral Regurgitation randomized trials demonstrated discordant results of transcatheter mitral valve repair in patients with secondary mitral regurgitation and symptomatic heart failure.
- Patients with higher severity of mitral regurgitation relative to left ventricular dilation derive greater symptom and mortality improvement from transcatheter mitral valve repair.
- Patient selection for transcatheter mitral valve repair requires evaluation by a multidisciplinary heart team in order to optimize patient outcomes.

INTRODUCTION

Secondary mitral regurgitation occurs in the absence of intrinsic mitral valve disease, most commonly due to ischemic or nonischemic cardiomyopathy. Given the prevalence of cardiomyopathy, secondary mitral regurgitation is more common than primary mitral regurgitation.[1] In ischemic cardiomyopathy, left ventricular remodeling/infarction/fibrosis leads to displacement of one or both papillary muscles. Regional left ventricular wall motion abnormalities lead to tethering and distortion of the mitral subvalvular apparatus and leaflet malcoaptation with subsequent mitral regurgitation. Whereas nonischemic cardiomyopathy results in a global ventricular dilation and increased sphericity. The papillary muscles are displaced apically and laterally, leading to leaflet tethering and distortion of the normally saddle-shaped mitral valve annulus. The distortion of the mitral valve annulus impairs leaflet coaptation leading to mitral regurgitation. As left ventricular function worsens and the ventricle dilates further, mitral regurgitation worsens.[2,3]

Among patients with heart failure with reduced ejection fraction, severe functional mitral regurgitation is a significant predictor of mortality after adjusting for patient demographics, left ventricular size, and function.[4] In a meta-analysis of 53 studies including 45,900 patients, the presence of any degree of secondary mitral regurgitation in patients with cardiomyopathy was associated with an increased risk of heart failure hospitalization, cardiac mortality, and all-cause mortality.[5]

Department of Cardiac Surgery, Michigan Medicine, University of Michigan, Ann Arbor, MI, USA
* Corresponding author. 1500 East Medical Center Drive, Ann Arbor, MI 48109.
E-mail address: mpienta@med.umich.edu

Cardiol Clin 41 (2023) 575–582
https://doi.org/10.1016/j.ccl.2023.06.008
0733-8651/23/© 2023 Elsevier Inc. All rights reserved.

Secondary mitral regurgitation is associated with higher all-cause mortality in both ischemic and nonischemic cardiomyopathy.[5] In patients with secondary mitral regurgitation due to ischemic cardiomyopathy, the presence of mitral regurgitation (MR) is associated with excess mortality independent of baseline characteristics and severity of left ventricular dysfunction.[6]

Secondary mitral regurgitation most commonly develops from left ventricular systolic dysfunction. Therefore, guideline-directed medical therapy (GDMT) aimed at improving LV function is the primary initial treatment modality for patients with secondary mitral regurgitation and reduced ejection fraction.[7,8] Implementation of GDMT has been demonstrated to decrease left ventricular volumes, reducing distortion of the mitral valve apparatus and improving secondary MR.[9] Improvements in mitral regurgitation have been demonstrated across multiple drug classes including renin-angiotensin-aldosterone blockers, beta-blockade, angiotensin-neprilysin inhibitors, and sodium glucose cotransporter inhibitors.[10–14]

There is limited current evidence to support surgical mitral valve repair in patients with severe secondary mitral regurgitation with reduced ejection fraction and persistent symptoms despite GDMT.[7] Several trials have shown symptomatic benefit for patients with coronary artery disease and ischemic cardiomyopathy who undergo mitral valve repair at the time of coronary artery bypass grafting.[15–17] Although these trials have not demonstrated a survival benefit, current guidelines recommend that it is reasonable to pursue mitral valve surgery at the time of coronary revascularization for ischemia.[7]

Transcatheter therapies have emerged as less-invasive treatments for secondary mitral regurgitation. In transcatheter edge-to-edge mitral valve repair, a device is placed to approximate the leading edge of the anterior and posterior mitral leaflets at the specified location, resulting in a double orifice valve. In essence, the transcatheter edge-to-edge repair replicates the Alfieri surgical mitral valve repair technique. The MitraClip (Abbott, Illinois, USA) has been the most widely adopted device.[18]

Current Evidence

Two recent randomized clinical trials, Percutaneous Repair with MitraClip for Severe Functional/Secondary Mitral Regurgitation (MITRA-FR) and Cardiovascular Outcomes Assessment of the MitraClip Percutaneous Therapy (COAPT) have evaluated the efficacy of transcatheter mitral valve repair in patients with severe secondary

mitral regurgitation and symptomatic heart failure with reduced ejection fraction. The MITRA-FR trial enrolled 304 patients with symptomatic heart failure with reduced ejection fraction and severe secondary mitral regurgitation at 37 centers in France. The patients were randomized in a 1:1 ratio to optimized medical therapy versus optimized medical therapy with percutaneous mitral valve repair with MitraClip.[19] Candidates for randomization had severe secondary MR defined as a regurgitant volume greater than 30 mL, effective regurgitant orifice area (EROA) greater than 20 mm², and LVEF 15% to 40%. Patients were excluded if they were candidates for mitral valve surgery as determined by local investigators. In MITRA-FR, the primary efficacy outcome was a composite of death from any cause or heart failure hospitalization at 1 year.

The COAPT trial randomized 614 patients with heart failure and moderate-to-severe or severe secondary mitral regurgitation on maximally tolerated GDMT in a 1:1 fashion to either medical therapy versus medical therapy plus transcatheter mitral valve repair.[20] Eligible patients had ischemic or nonischemic cardiomyopathy with LVEF 20% to 50%, grade 3+ or 4+ secondary mitral regurgitation, and had heart failure symptoms (NYHA II-IVa) despite maximal GDMT and cardiac resynchronization therapy, if indicated. In COAPT, mod–severe or severe secondary MR was defined as EROA greater than 30 mm,² regurgitant volume greater than 45 mL, and LVEF 20% to 50%. Assessment by the heart team determined that patients were not appropriate for mitral valve surgery. The primary effectiveness endpoint was heart failure hospitalizations in 2 years of follow-up.

DISCUSSION

Despite evaluating the same device, the results of MITRA-FR and COAPT were discordant. MITRA-FR demonstrated no benefit from GDMT with transcatheter mitral valve repair at 12 months compared with GDMT alone (all-cause death or heart failure hospitalization; intervention 54.6% vs control 51.3%, odds ratio 1.16 [95% CI: 0.73–1.84] P = .53). COAPT demonstrated lower all-cause mortality (29.1% vs 46.1%, hazard ratio 0.62, P < .001) and lower rate of hospitalizations (35.8% vs 67.9% per patient-year, hazard ratio 0.53, P < .0001) at 2 years in patients treated with MitraClip compared with GDMT alone. In COAPT, the benefits of MitraClip implantation were present across categories of NYHA classification, with consistently reduced rates of heart failure hospitalization ambulatory NYHA functional class IV (40.9% vs 78.3%; HR: 0.34; 95% CI: 0.14–0.86); NYHA functional class III (35.9% vs 55.6%; HR: 0.53; 95% CI: 0.37–0.76); and NYHA functional class II (33.0% vs 51.3%; HR: 0.57; 95% CI: 0.38–0.86).[21]

Although the trails were similar, there were key factors that may explain the differences in trial outcomes. Overall, the COAPT trial had more stringent inclusion/exclusion criteria with limits on left ventricular size (left ventricular end systolic diameter <70 mm) and exclusion of patients with evidence of right heart failure or pulmonary hypertension. Therefore, patients included in COAPT had a notably smaller average indexed left ventricular end diastolic volume (LVEDV) compared with patients included in MITRA-FR (101 ± 34 mL/m^2 vs 135 ± 35 mL/m^2).[19,20] This difference would suggest that the MITRA-FR patients with larger LV end-diastolic volume had a more advanced stage of LV disease.

MITRA-FR also used less restrictive 2012 European Society of Cardiology guidelines (EROA >20 mm^2) to define severe mitral regurgitation resulting in a patient population with smaller effective regurgitant area (0.31 ± 0.10 mm^2 vs 0.41 ± 0.15 mm^2); therefore, the patients in MITRA-FR had less-severe MR than those treated in COAPT. Additionally, the COAPT trial was notably more selective when evaluating patients for inclusion with 57.8% (911/1576) of patients screened and deemed ineligible compared with 32% (145/452) in Mitra-FR. There were fewer procedural complications in the COAPT trial (8.5%) compared with MITRA-FR (14.6%). Patients in both MITRA-FR and COAPT achieved similar early reductions in mitral regurgitation to 2+ or less with 91.9% and 95.0% of patients, respectively.

Additionally, although both COAPT and MITRA-FR required the treatment and control groups to continue GDMT for heart failure, the medical management of patients differed between the 2 trials. In order to be eligible for the COAPT trial, patients were required to be on maximally tolerated GDMT (as adjudicated by a central eligibility committee) and to have undergone cardiac resynchronization therapy if appropriate. Additionally, utilization rates for specific medication classes and medications changes were recorded throughout the trial for both the treatment and control groups. Conversely, in the MITRA-FR trial, medical therapy was not optimized in all patients at baseline and adequacy of GDMT was assessed by local investigators at each site. The rates of utilization of each class of drug recommended as part of GDMT were not recorded throughout the MITRA-FR trial. Notably, a larger proportion of patients in MITRA-FR was treated with renin-angiotensin blockade and was more likely to be treated with a neprilysin inhibitor.[19,20] the medical management in MITRA-FR may more closely resemble real world practice given that decisions regarding titration/optimization were left to local investigators. Titration of GDMT medications during the trial may have reduced secondary mitral regurgitation and attenuated the potential additional benefit of transcatheter mitral repair.

The discordant results of COAPT and MITRA-FR have subsequently been redemonstrated in follow-up studies. Recently, the COAPT investigators published 36-month outcomes, including a subgroup analysis of patients originally assigned to the control group and only treated with GDMT who then were allowed to crossover and undergo MitraClip.[22] Three-year outcomes were available in 92.4% eligible patients in the GDMT plus MitraClip arm and in 87.4% patients in the GDMT-alone arm. The benefits of MitraClip evident at 24 months in the initial trial were also apparent at 36 months, with all-cause mortality (42.8% vs 55.5%, $P < .001$) and heart failure hospitalizations (46.5% vs 81.5%, $P < .0001$) lower in the MitraClip group. Among 58 patients (18.6%) initially treated in the GDMT-alone control arm who subsequently underwent MitraClip, there was a lower incidence of heart failure hospitalization and the composite of death or heart failure hospitalization compared with patients who continued on medical therapy alone. Additionally, the 2-year results for the Mitra-FR were recently published, which continued to demonstrate no difference in the primary outcome (composite of all-cause death and unplanned hospitalization) between the treatment and control groups (63.8% vs 67.1%).[23]

Health Status After Transcatheter Mitral Valve Repair in Cardiovascular Outcomes Assessment of the MitraClip Percutaneous Therapy

A subanalysis of the COAPT trial evaluated patients' symptoms and quality of life using the Kansas City Cardiomyopathy Questionnaire (KCCQ) and the Medical Outcomes Study Short-Form 36 Health Survey, physical summary score (SF-36 PCS) and mental summary scores. Among patients who underwent MitraClip, the KCCQ increased at 1 month compared with patients in the control arm with KCCQ mean difference 15.9 points; 95% CI 12.3 to 19.5 points, $P < .001$. Similarly, the SF-36 PCS and MCS scores also improved in the MitraClip group, with the mean difference between groups of 5.3 points (95% CI: 3.8–6.8 points) and 5.2 points (95% CI: 3.3–7.1 points), respectively. Among surviving patients, the symptomatic benefits were sustained at both 12 and 24 months.[24] The largest improvements in KCCQ scores were observed in patients who underwent MitraClip who were in NYHA functional class III or ambulatory class IV at baseline.[21]

Extension to Real World Data

Subsequent studies have extended the findings from COAPT and MITRA-FR to real-world registry data. A recent analysis of the European Registry of Transcatheter Repair for Secondary Mitral Regurgitation (EuroSMR) identified 1022 patients treated with transcatheter mitral repair between 2008 and 2019 and stratified them into groups based on eligibility for COAPT (eligible [n = 353 (34.5%)] and ineligible [n = 669 (65.5%)]) and MITRA-FR (eligible [n = 408 (48.3%)] and ineligible [n = 437 (51.7%)]).[25] Stratification of patients according to MITRA-FR eligibility criteria demonstrated overall similar outcomes to the MITRA-FR trial, with no difference in all-cause mortality ($P = .19$). However, when patients were stratified according to COAPT enrollment criteria, patients who were COAPT-eligible demonstrated lower all-cause mortality than those patients who were COAPT-ineligible ($P < .001$). Similarly, a retrospective study of 304 patients with secondary mitral regurgitation undergoing MitraClip in 3 Italian centers demonstrated that patients with a COAPT-like profile have a better prognosis than patients who would have met exclusion criteria for the COAPT trial.[26] Similar results were observed in a single-center retrospective French study.[27] In a single-center German study of 458 patients undergoing MitraClip for secondary mitral regurgitation with median follow-up of 5 years, patients with less than 1+ mitral regurgitation at discharge had higher survival than patients with higher grades of MR at discharge.[28]

Proportionate and Disproportionate Mitral Regurgitation

Subsequent to the publication of the discordant results of MITRA-FR and COAPT, a new conceptual framework regarding classification of "proportionate" and "disproportionate" mitral regurgitation was introduced to explain the findings.[29] In this conceptual framework, the proportionality of secondary mitral regurgitation is determined by the relationship/ratio between effective regurgitant area (EROA) and left ventricular dilation (LVEDV). Mitral regurgitation is deemed disproportionate if the magnitude of regurgitant flow is greater than would be expected based on the left ventricular volume (dilation). Proportionate mitral regurgitation develops from symmetric tethering of the mitral valve leaflets secondary to left ventricular dilation (low EROA/LVEDV). Disproportionate mitral regurgitation is associated with local wall motion abnormalities (left bundle branch block, regional fibrosis, aneurysm, and so forth) causing asymmetric or eccentric mitral regurgitation that is more severe than can be explained purely by overall left ventricular dilation (high EROA/LVEDV).

Packer and Grayburn have suggested that disproportionate MR is present when EROA/LVEDV is greater than 0.14 (**Fig. 1**).[30] For example, a patient with EROA of 0.3 cm^2 but with LVEDV of 160 mL would have more mitral regurgitation than would be expected by left ventricular volume.[29] According to this framework, therapies directed at reducing left ventricular dilation/volume, such as neurohormonal antagonists (as part of GDMT regimen), show benefit for patients with

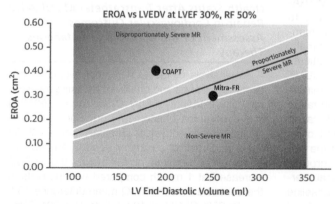

Fig. 1. Relationship between EROA and LVEDV illustrating domains that define disproportionately severe, proportionately severe, and nonsevere functional mitral regurgitation. The diagram depicts the relation between EROA and LVEDV, assuming an LVEF of 30% with a regurgitant fraction of 50%. The blue line represents the hypothetical relationship when the degree of severe MR is proportional to the LVEDV. The gray area approximates a degree of uncertainty that is determined by the imprecision inherent in the measurement of EROA as well as the hemodynamic state of the patient. The pink area in the upper left depicts severe MR that is disproportionate to LV dilation. The green area in the lower right depicts nonsevere MR. The average patient enrolled in the MITRA-FR and COAPT trials is shown by the red dots, based on the information made public to date. (*From* Grayburn PA, Sannino A, Packer M. Proportionate and Disproportionate Functional Mitral Regurgitation: A New Conceptual Framework That Reconciles the Results of the MITRA-FR and COAPT Trials. JACC Cardiovasc Imaging. 2019;12(2):353-362.)

proportionate MR because these treatments aim to reduce left ventricular volume/dilation. Additionally, treatments that aim to treat the components of the mitral valve (transcatheter mitral valve repair or replacement) are beneficial for patients with disproportionate MR.

Applying the proportionality framework to the COAPT and MITRA-FR studies, there were notable differences in LVEDV and EROA between the 2 studies (LVEDV index: COAPT 101 ± 34 mL/m^2 vs MITRA-FR 135 ± 35 mL/m^2; EROA: COAPT 0.41 ± 0.15 mm^2 vs MITRA-FR 0.31 ± 0.10 mm^2).[19,20] The COAPT trial included patients with larger EROA than MITRA-FR but smaller LVEDV. Patients with higher EROA relative to LVEDV (disproportionate MR), such as those patients included in COAPT, benefit from transcatheter mitral valve repair because the degree of mitral regurgitation is larger than would be expected based on left ventricular dimensions alone. Reanalysis of the COAPT patient cohort into subgroups based on EROA and LVEDV index demonstrated that the efficacy of transcatheter mitral valve repair in the subgroup of patients with proportionate MR (LVEDV index >96 mL/m^2 and EROA ≤30 mm^2) was similar to the outcomes of MITRA-FR.[30,31]

Although the concept of MR proportionality is an intuitive and appealing framework, the model has not been able to fully explain differences in outcome after transcatheter mitral valve repair. Reanalysis of the MITRA-FR trial according to the proportionality framework identified a subset of patients with disproportionate MR; however, these patients did not benefit from transcatheter mitral valve repair.[32] These results challenge the generalizability/applicability of the proportionality framework. However, it is possible that differences in management of GDMT during the 2 randomized clinical trials may account for these findings.

An analysis of 1016 patients in the EuroSMR registry demonstrated that all patients treated with transcatheter mitral repair had symptomatic improvement, regardless of EROA/LVEDV.[33] However, there was no difference in mortality after transcatheter mitral valve repair among patients with proportionate and disproportionate MR. Secondary mitral regurgitation is dynamic and varies with loading conditions, which may alter measurements of EROA, LVEF, and LVEDV over time and cause the proportionality to vary in a given patient.[34]

Cost-Effectiveness of Transcatheter Mitral Valve Repair

Among patients with symptomatic heart failure and severe secondary mitral regurgitation, transcatheter mitral valve repair increases life expectancy and quality of life compared with GDMT at an incremental cost of about US$45,000 per patient. Overall treatment costs at 2 years are approximately US$35,000 higher for patients undergoing transcatheter repair compared with those undergoing medical treatment alone, which is attributable largely to the initial procedural cost. However, follow-up medical care costs were reduced by US$11,690 per patient with transcatheter mitral valve repair versus GDMT (95% CI, −US$20,714 to −US$3010; P = .018).[35] The largest relative cost savings were attributable to a reduction in heart failure hospitalizations among patients undergoing Mitra-Clip. The incremental cost-effectiveness ratio for transcatheter mitral valve repair was US$55,600, which compares favorably to other interventions in the United States, including transcatheter aortic valve replacement.[36] Three-year data for the COAPT trial demonstrated a greater absolute benefit in reductions of death or heart failure hospitalization for transcatheter mitral valve repair compared with GDMT alone, suggesting that the cost-effectiveness of transcatheter mitral valve repair with improve with longer term data. Additional analyses of cost-effectiveness in real-world patients outside of clinical trials are required.

MitraClip and Heart Transplantation

Transcatheter mitral valve repair has been evaluated as a bridging strategy for patients with heart failure who may be heart transplant candidates. The MitraBridge Registry followed 119 patients with moderate-to-severe or severe mitral regurgitation and advanced heart failure undergoing MitraClip, of which 26% were listed for heart transplant and the remainder were bridge to decision or bridge to candidacy. There were no perioperative deaths (30-day mortality 0%).[37] About 60.5% of patients achieved at least one NYHA functional class improvement and 23.5% of patients had significant clinical improvement such that they no longer had an indication for heart transplantation. The COAPT trial demonstrated that fewer patients who underwent MitraClip placement proceeded to heart transplant than those treated with medical therapy (3.0% vs 7.1%, P = .02).[20] However, the COAPT trial was not powered to determine a difference in progression to heart transplant or left ventricular assist device when patients were stratified by NYHA class.[21]

Guidelines

The Food and Drug Administration has approved the MitraClip in the United States for secondary mitral regurgitation based on the results of the COAPT trial. Similarly, current American College of Cardiology (ACC)/American Heart Association (AHA) guidelines state that transcatheter edge-to-edge mitral valve repair is reasonable in patients with symptomatic heart failure with chronic severe secondary MR while on optimal GDMT, in cases where LVEF 20% to 50%, left ventricular end systolic diameter of 70 millimeters (mm) or greater, and pulmonary artery systolic pressure of 70 mm Hg or lesser.[7,8] The European Society of Cardiology (ESC)/European Association for Cardio-Thoracic Surgery (EACTS) guidelines were also updated to recommend that transcatheter mitral valve repair be considered in patients with heart failure and severe secondary mitral regurgitation who are receiving optimal medical therapy and are as close as possible to fulfilling COAPT eligibility criteria.[38]

Patient Selection

Appropriate patient selection is essential to determining those patients that will benefit from transcatheter edge-to-edge mitral valve repair. A multidisciplinary heart team is paramount when evaluating these patients to not only determine which patients are appropriate for intervention but also to guide appropriate medical optimization and timing of the procedure. These teams should incorporate standardized methods/frameworks for patient evaluation and incorporate clinicians with expertise in surgery, heart failure, structural heart interventions, and imaging.[39] Additionally, sonographic expertise is required to determine the severity of secondary mitral regurgitation and to ensure patients are anatomically appropriate for intervention. Surgical consultation is critical to determine eligibility for surgical intervention and if additional or alternative interventions would provide symptomatic or survival benefit to the patients (coronary artery bypass grafting, multivalve procedures, Maze procedure, left atrial appendage ligation, left ventricular assist device/heart transplant).

Several risk scores have been developed to assist with patient selection for transcatheter mitral valve repair. The COAPT Risk Score was derived from the COAPT trial cohort and includes 8 clinical, echocardiographic, and treatment variables and provides modest ability (C statistical = 0.74) to discriminate outcomes among patients with heart failure and secondary mitral regurgitation, although no validation cohort was used.[40] The MitraScore and MITRALITY models were derived from multi-institutional registries including patients with primary and secondary MR undergoing transcatheter mitral valve repair and also generated moderate discriminatory capacity in validation cohorts of patients with functional MR (Mitrascore AUC = 0.65, MITRALITY AUC = 0.77).[41,42]

FUTURE DIRECTIONS

The RESHAPE-HF Trial [A Randomized Study of the MitraClip Device in Heart Failure Patients With Clinically Significant Functional Mitral Regurgitation (NCT01772108)] will provide additional information regarding the utility of transcatheter mitral valve repair in patients with heart failure and secondary mitral regurgitation treated with GDMT.

SUMMARY

Initial management of patients with secondary mitral regurgitation and heart failure requires optimization of GDMT. A heart team approach should be used in the care of these complex patients. The concept of mitral regurgitation proportionality, as determined by the EROA/LVEDV ratio, may further guide decisions regarding which patients may benefit from transcatheter intervention. Current evidence suggests that transcatheter mitral valve repair has a role as a useful adjunct to GDMT in select patients with symptomatic heart failure with reduced ejection fraction and severe secondary mitral regurgitation who fulfill COAPT-eligibility criteria. However, there are limited data to guide utilization of transcatheter mitral valve therapies in patients with advanced heart failure. Additional studies are needed to clarify which patients with advanced heart failure would benefit from transcatheter mitral valve repair.

CLINICS CARE POINTS

- Transcatheter mitral valve repair provides symptomatic and survival benefit in select patients with symptomatic heart failure and severe secondary mitral regurgitation despite optimization of GDMT.

- Current selection criteria for transcatheter mitral valve repair in secondary mitral regurgitation are based on the inclusion criteria of the COAPT trial: LVEF 20% to 50%, LVEDD less than 7 cm, pulmonary artery systolic pressure less than 70 mm Hg, and symptomatic heart failure (NYHA class II-IV) despite medical optimization.

DISCLOSURES

M.J. Pienta: No Disclosures. M.A. Romano: No Disclosures.

REFERENCES

1. de Marchena E, Badiye A, Robalino G, et al. Respective prevalence of the different carpentier classes of mitral regurgitation: a stepping stone for future therapeutic research and development. J Card Surg 2011;26(4):385–92.

2. Scotti A, Margonato A, Godino C. Percutaneous mitral valve repair in patients with secondary mitral regurgitation and advanced heart failure. Mini-invasive Surgery 2020;2020. https://doi.org/10.20517/2574-1225.2020.38.

3. Asgar AW, Mack MJ, Stone GW. Secondary mitral regurgitation in heart failure: pathophysiology, prognosis, and therapeutic considerations. J Am Coll Cardiol 2015;65(12):1231–48.

4. Goliasch G, Bartko PE, Pavo N, et al. Refining the prognostic impact of functional mitral regurgitation in chronic heart failure. Eur Heart J 2018;39(1):39–46.

5. Sannino A, Smith RL 2nd, Schiattarella GG, et al. Survival and cardiovascular outcomes of patients with secondary mitral regurgitation: a systematic review and meta-analysis. JAMA Cardiol 2017;2(10):1130–9.

6. Grigioni F, Enriquez-Sarano M, Zehr KJ, et al. Ischemic mitral regurgitation: long-term outcome and prognostic implications with quantitative Doppler assessment. Circulation 2001;103(13):1759–64.

7. Otto CM, Nishimura RA, Bonow RO, et al. 2020 ACC/AHA guideline for the management of patients with valvular heart disease: a report of the American college of cardiology/American heart association joint committee on clinical practice guidelines. J Am Coll Cardiol 2021;77(4):e25–197.

8. Heidenreich PA, Bozkurt B, Aguilar D, et al. 2022 AHA/ACC/HFSA guideline for the management of heart failure: a report of the american college of cardiology/american heart association joint committee on clinical practice guidelines. J Am Coll Cardiol 2022;79(17):e263–421.

9. Milwidsky A, Mathai SV, Topilsky Y, et al. Medical therapy for functional mitral regurgitation. Circ Heart Fail 2022;15(9):e009689.

10. Kang DH, Park SJ, Shin SH, et al. Angiotensin receptor neprilysin inhibitor for functional mitral regurgitation. Circulation 2019;139(11):1354–65.

11. Nasser R, Van Assche L, Vorlat A, et al. Evolution of functional mitral regurgitation and prognosis in medically managed heart failure patients with reduced ejection fraction. JACC Heart Fail 2017;5(9):652–9.

12. Comin-Colet J, Sanchez-Corral MA, Manito N, et al. Effect of carvedilol therapy on functional mitral regurgitation, ventricular remodeling, and contractility in patients with heart failure due to left ventricular systolic dysfunction. Transplant Proc 2002;34:177–8.

13. Zannad F, Ferreira JP, Pocock SJ, et al. SGLT2 inhibitors in patients with heart failure with reduced ejection fraction: a meta-analysis of the EMPEROR-Reduced and DAPA-HF trials. Lancet 2020;396(10254):819–29.

14. Lee MMY, Brooksbank KJM, Wetherall K, et al. Effect of empagliflozin on left ventricular volumes in patients with type 2 diabetes, or prediabetes, and heart failure with reduced ejection fraction (SUGAR-DM-HF). Circulation 2021;143(6):516–25.

15. Fattouch K, Guccione F, Sampognaro R, et al. POINT: efficacy of adding mitral valve restrictive annuloplasty to coronary artery bypass grafting in patients with moderate ischemic mitral valve regurgitation: a randomized trial. J Thorac Cardiovasc Surg 2009;138(2):278–85.

16. Chan KMJ, Punjabi PP, Flather M, et al. Coronary artery bypass surgery with or without mitral valve annuloplasty in moderate functional ischemic mitral regurgitation: final results of the Randomized Ischemic Mitral Evaluation (RIME) trial. Circulation 2012;126(21):2502–10.

17. Cheitlin MD. Impact of mitral valve annuloplasty combined with revascularization in patients with functional ischemic mitral regurgitation. Year Bk Cardiol 2008;2008:420–4.

18. Mack M, Carroll JD, Thourani V, et al. Transcatheter mitral valve therapy in the United States: a report from the STS-ACC TVT registry. J Am Coll Cardiol 2021;78(23):2326–53.

19. Obadia JF, Messika-Zeitoun D, Leurent G, et al. Percutaneous repair or medical treatment for secondary mitral regurgitation. N Engl J Med 2018;379(24):2297–306.

20. Stone GW, Lindenfeld J, Abraham WT, et al. Transcatheter mitral-valve repair in patients with heart failure. N Engl J Med 2018;379(24):2307–18.

21. Giustino G, Lindenfeld J, Abraham WT, et al. NYHA functional classification and outcomes after transcatheter mitral valve repair in heart failure: the COAPT trial. JACC Cardiovasc Interv 2020;13(20):2317–28.

22. Mack MJ, Lindenfeld J, Abraham WT, et al. 3-year outcomes of transcatheter mitral valve repair in patients with heart failure. J Am Coll Cardiol 2021;77(8):1029–40.

23. Iung B, Armoiry X, Vahanian A, et al. Percutaneous repair or medical treatment for secondary mitral regurgitation: outcomes at 2 years. Eur J Heart Fail 2019;21(12):1619–27.

24. Arnold SV, Chinnakondepalli KM, Spertus JA, et al. Health status after transcatheter mitral-valve repair

in heart failure and secondary mitral regurgitation: COAPT trial. J Am Coll Cardiol 2019;73(17): 2123–32.

25. Koell B, Orban M, Weimann J, et al. Outcomes stratified by adapted inclusion criteria after mitral edge-to-edge repair. J Am Coll Cardiol 2021;78(24): 2408–21.

26. Adamo M, Fiorelli F, Melica B, et al. COAPT-like profile predicts long-term outcomes in patients with secondary mitral regurgitation undergoing MitraClip implantation. JACC Cardiovasc Interv 2021;14(1): 15–25.

27. Iliadis C, Metze C, Körber MI, et al. Impact of COAPT trial exclusion criteria in real-world patients undergoing transcatheter mitral valve repair. Int J Cardiol 2020;316:189–94.

28. Reichart D, Kalbacher D, Rübsamen N, et al. The impact of residual mitral regurgitation after MitraClip therapy in functional mitral regurgitation. Eur J Heart Fail 2020;22(10):1840–8.

29. Grayburn PA, Sannino A, Packer M. Proportionate and disproportionate functional mitral regurgitation: a new conceptual framework that reconciles the results of the MITRA-FR and COAPT trials. JACC Cardiovasc Imaging 2019;12(2):353–62.

30. Packer M, Grayburn PA. New evidence supporting a novel conceptual framework for distinguishing proportionate and disproportionate functional mitral regurgitation. JAMA Cardiol 2020;5(4):469–75.

31. Lindenfeld J, Abraham WT, Grayburn PA, et al. Association of effective regurgitation orifice area to left ventricular end-diastolic volume ratio with transcatheter mitral valve repair outcomes: a secondary analysis of the COAPT trial. JAMA cardiology 2021;6(4):427–36.

32. Messika-Zeitoun D, Iung B, Armoiry X, et al. Impact of mitral regurgitation severity and left ventricular remodeling on outcome after mitraclip implantation: results from the mitra-fr trial. JACC Cardiovasc Imaging 2021;14(4):742–52.

33. Orban M, Karam N, Lubos E, et al. Impact of proportionality of secondary mitral regurgitation on outcome after transcatheter mitral valve repair. JACC Cardiovasc Imaging 2021;14(4):715–25.

34. Grayburn PA, Packer M, Sannino A, et al. Disproportionate secondary mitral regurgitation: myths, misconceptions and clinical implications. Heart 2020. https://doi.org/10.1136/heartjnl-2020-316992.

35. Baron SJ, Wang K, Arnold SV, et al. Cost-effectiveness of transcatheter mitral valve repair versus medical therapy in patients with heart failure and secondary mitral regurgitation: results from the COAPT trial. Circulation 2019;140(23):1881–91.

36. Reynolds MR, Lei Y, Wang K, et al. Cost-effectiveness of transcatheter aortic valve replacement with a self-expanding prosthesis versus surgical aortic valve replacement. J Am Coll Cardiol 2016;67(1): 29–38.

37. Godino C, Munafò A, Scotti A, et al. MitraClip in secondary mitral regurgitation as a bridge to heart transplantation: 1-year outcomes from the International MitraBridge Registry. J Heart Lung Transplant 2020;39(12):1353–62.

38. Vahanian A, Beyersdorf F, Praz F, et al. 2021 ESC/EACTS guidelines for the management of valvular heart disease: developed by the task force for the management of valvular heart disease of the european society of cardiology (ESC) and the European association for Cardio-Thoracic surgery (EACTS). Revista Española de Cardiología (English Edition) 2022;75(6):524. https://doi.org/10.1016/j.rec.2022.05.006.

39. Coats AJS, Anker SD, Baumbach A, et al. The management of secondary mitral regurgitation in patients with heart failure: a joint position statement from the heart failure association (HFA), European association of cardiovascular imaging (EACVI), European heart Rhythm association (EHRA), and European association of percutaneous cardiovascular interventions (EAPCI) of the ESC. Eur Heart J 2021;42(13):1254–69.

40. Shah N, Madhavan MV, Gray WA, et al. Prediction of death or HF hospitalization in patients with severe FMR: the COAPT risk score. JACC Cardiovasc Interv 2022;15(19):1893–905.

41. Raposeiras-Roubin S, Adamo M, Freixa X, et al. A score to assess mortality after percutaneous mitral valve repair. J Am Coll Cardiol 2022;79(6):562–73.

42. Zweck E, Spieker M, Horn P, et al. Machine learning identifies clinical parameters to predict mortality in patients undergoing transcatheter mitral valve repair. JACC Cardiovasc Interv 2021;14(18): 2027–36.

Guide to Temporary Mechanical Support in Cardiogenic Shock
Choosing Wisely

David Snipelisky, MD*, Jerry D. Estep, MD

KEYWORDS

- Cardiogenic shock • Advanced heart failure • Temporary mechanical circulatory support

KEY POINTS

- Owing to the acuity of cardiogenic shock and high mortality rate, the use of temporary mechanical circulatory support has increased significantly over the past decade.
- It is important to utilize a multidisciplinary approach, including shock teams, when deciding on the candidacy for temporary mechanical circulatory support.
- Defining the phenotype of cardiogenic shock is key to aiding in the selection of support devices.
- A wide array of temporary mechanical circulatory support devices exist, each with its own hemodynamic blueprint.
- Continuous assessments of cardiac function are key to understanding a patient's "exit strategy" as well as assess candidacy for either device weaning or further escalation in therapy.

INTRODUCTION

As a multiorgan pathology with a mortality rate of up to 60%, cardiogenic shock is a state of circulatory failure in which the heart is unable to pump sufficient amount of oxygenated blood to meet the metabolic demands of the body.[1–4] Cardiogenic shock can occur secondary to either ischemic or nonischemic causes, and treatment may be guided based on the inherent etiology. Pharmacotherapies to treat this pathologic state include inotropes and vasopressors, yet these drugs can increase the myocardial oxygen consumption and decrease tissue perfusion, ultimately creating an environment unfavorable to a potentially failing heart.[1,5,6] With acute myocardial infarction, the most common cause of cardiogenic shock and occurring in approximately two-third of patients, an increase in patients with nonischemic etiologies has been more apparent over the past decade owing to the higher prevalence of refractory heart failure, with 5% of all hospitalized patients having end-stage disease.[1,5,7,8]

Following recognition of cardiogenic shock, in most circumstances, the first steps in management include selecting appropriate pharmacotherapies and very closely monitoring clinical response. Although pharmacotherapy can be successful, a significant portion of patients with cardiogenic shock have a pathology refractory to drug therapy[1,5,9,10] (**Fig. 1**). In these patients, more aggressive therapies such as temporary mechanical circulatory support (tMCS) may be required. The field of tMCS has evolved tremendously, with the first reports of left heart assist devices stemming from the mid-1970s among patients who could not be successfully weaned from cardiopulmonary bypass to full biventricular support with configurations allowing for patients to be fully ambulatory in the more contemporary time period.[1,2,9]

Robert and Suzanne Tomsich Department of Cardiology, Section of Heart Failure & Cardiac Transplant Medicine, Cleveland Clinic, 2950 Cleveland Clinic Boulevard, Weston, FL 33331, USA
* Corresponding author.
E-mail address: snipeld@ccf.org

Cardiol Clin 41 (2023) 583–592
https://doi.org/10.1016/j.ccl.2023.06.004

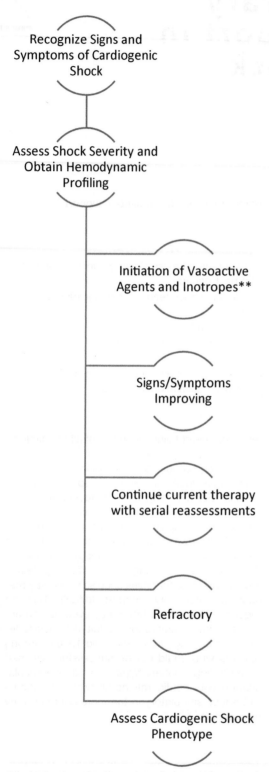

Fig. 1. Shock recognition and initial management algorithm. ** assuming temporary mechanical circulatory support not needed.

Once the need for tMCS has been defined, most programs use shock teams to evaluate in a multidisciplinary fashion (**Fig. 2**). Decision-making includes discussions of the type of tMCS to utilize, as delineated by the phenotype of shock.[1,10–12] Furthermore, it is important to understand the "destination" of tMCS—whether the goal is for recovery, as a bridge to more durable advanced therapies such as durable left ventricular assist devices, or cardiac transplantation.[13] In addition, discussions should be regarding whether the ability to bridge a patient to a certain destination is feasible taking into account other comorbidities, noncardiac end-organ manifestations, and patient goals of care, therefore ensuring a so-called "exit strategy."[1]

Among patients necessitating the need for tMCS, it is important to understand the cardiogenic shock phenotype as this allows for a better understanding of the type of support needed.[1,5] A wide array of devices are available, each with its own hemodynamic blueprint, and understanding whether a patient requires left, right, or biventricular support is key[1,11] (**Fig. 3**). In addition, it is important to realize that a patient's hemodynamic profile and hemodynamic requirements may change over time, reflecting the need to be fluid in support selection.[1,2]

LEFT VENTRICLE SUPPORT SYSTEMS
Intra-aortic Balloon Pump

The intra-aortic balloon pump (IABP) is among the oldest available tMCS options and the most commonly used one today. First described in the 1960s, this support option operates by inflating a helium-filled balloon positioned in the descending

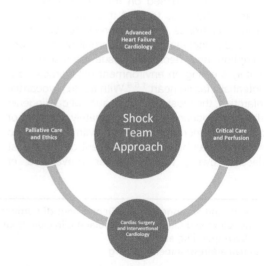

Fig. 2. Multidisciplinary shock team components.

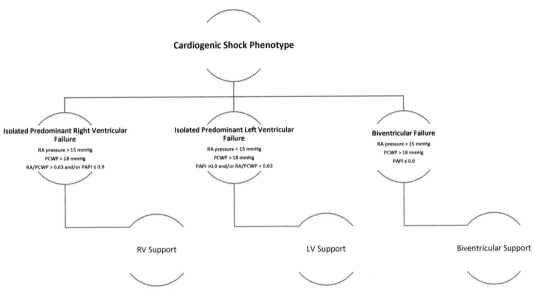

Fig. 3. Different cardiogenic shock phenotypes.

aorta during diastole and deflating during systole, allowing for improved myocardial oxygen delivery and coronary perfusion through counterpulsation (**Fig. 4**).[1,5,7,9,10,12,14] A key factor to ensure maximal benefit with IABP support is appropriate timing of the inflation and deflation of the balloon which can be observed on a display console that provides continuous waveform pressure tracings. Either by paralleling the balloon counterpulsation with the electrocardiogram tracing or an arterial pressure waveform obtained from the arterial lumen of the IABP catheter, appropriate timing of inflation and deflation can be confirmed.[1,5]

The hemodynamic effect of IABP therapy provides a relatively small increase in cardiac output by approximately 0.5 L/min yet also decreases afterload which helps to further decrease the left ventricular end-diastolic pressure. This ultimately decreases myocardial oxygen consumption while increasing myocardial and coronary oxygen delivery.[1,5,7,9,10,12,14] Positioned distal to the left subclavian artery, the IABP can generally be placed via either the femoral or axillary artery. In the axillary artery configuration, patients are usually able to ambulate, which holds value among those for whom longer duration of support is anticipated. The largest single-center experience of 195 patients demonstrated the feasibility and safety of axillary artery placement, with 120 of those patients supported until heart transplantation.[15] Important complications with IABP include vascular complications such as bleeding, limb ischemia, and renal ischemia. In patients with severe aortic regurgitation, IABP is not recommended as the degree of regurgitation may increase,

and IABP implantation should be carefully evaluated among patients with a severe peripheral arterial disease.[1,5,7,9,10,12,14]

As with the other tMCS options, data regarding IABP use are mixed with a gap between frequency of use and current clinical guidance.[1,5,7,9,10,12,14] The IABP-SHOCK II trial failed to demonstrate improvement in 30-day and 1-year survival among patients with IABP therapy, yet patients with IABP therapy tended to be quite ill, with almost half having required resuscitation before IABP placement and almost all supported by high-dose vasoactive medications at the time of IABP placement.[16] At present, IABP use is a class IIb recommendation by the American College of Cardiology/American Heart Association primarily based on registry data.[10]

Impella

As a series of devices of varying support, the Impella (Abiomed, Danvers, MA, USA) continuous flow microaxial pump functions based on the Archimedes screw principle in which blood is delivered into the aorta by exerting negative pressure on the propeller tip that moves blood from the left ventricle through the inlet and Impella cannula (**Fig. 5**).[5] This allows for direct left ventricle unloading.[1,5] The Impella devices allow for partial or full hemodynamic support for the left ventricule. Support levels vary, with devices allowing for cardiac output augmentation by up to 2.5 L/min (Impella 2.5), 3 to 4 L/min (Impella CP), 5 L/min (Impella 5.0), and up to 6 L/min (Impella 5.5). Both the Impella 5.0 and Impella 5.5 are generally surgically

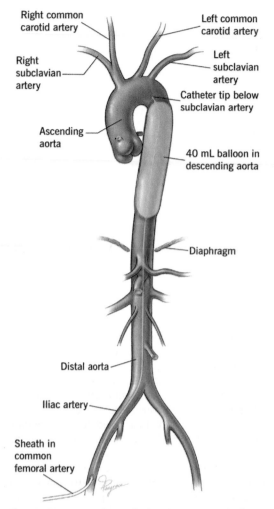

Right common carotid artery

Left common carotid artery

Right subclavian artery

Left subclavian artery

Catheter tip below subclavian artery

Ascending aorta

40 mL balloon in descending aorta

Diaphragm

Distal aorta

Iliac artery

Sheath in common femoral artery

Fig. 4. Demonstration of the intra-aortic balloon pump in the descending aorta. (Reprinted with permission, Cleveland Clinic Foundation ©2023. All Rights Reserved.)

placed devices.[5] Although IABP is still the most commonly utilized tMCS device, recent data demonstrate increasing utilization of Impella devices.[17]

By directly unloading the left ventricle, the Impella devices are able to immediately lower the left ventricular end-diastolic pressure, ultimately decreasing myocardial consumption. Left ventricular wall tension is also reduced. As blood is diverted into the ascending aorta, the increase in forward flow can further augment the mean arterial pressure aiding in tissue perfusion. The device power levels can be adjusted to augment the amount of blood removed from the left ventricle.[1,5,7,9,10,12,14] Although evidence regarding Impella support is limited to observational data, one large series describes a total of 236 patients supported by an

Impella 5.0 actively listed for transplant, with the majority bridged to either heart transplantation or durable left-ventricular assist device support. Among this cohort, the median time of support was 13 days, and posttransplant complications related to Impella use were rare.[18]

Similar to the IABP, the Impella devices can be placed in either the femoral artery or axillary artery positions. With the axillary position, patients can ambulate. All patients should be anticoagulated, and correct device positioning across the aortic valve is key to ensure appropriate function.[5] It is important to confirm that the cannula does not abut the anterior mitral valve leaflet as this can result in functional mitral valve stenosis. Complication rates are higher with Impella support than with IABP and include hemolysis as a result of mechanical shearing of blood cells, which can subsequently lead to kidney injury and anemia. This needs to be monitored closely, particularly among patients listed for heart transplantation for whom renal failure and blood transfusions carry postoperative risk. Hemolysis is generally not as severe with the larger cannula sizes. Other complications include thrombus within the cannula, vascular complications, limb ischemia, and infection. The presence of a peripheral arterial disease increases such risks.[1,5,14]

TandemHeart

An extracorporeal, centrifugal continuous flow pump, the TandemHeart (LivaNova, UK) operates by diverting blood from the left atrium to the systemic arterial circulation. It is able to decrease the left ventricle end diastolic pressure by venting the left atrium while also decreasing cardiac work and myocardial oxygen demand. This pump is placed by a trans-septal puncture in which a cannula is positioned within the left atrium with blood flow returning to the femoral artery and can provide support of up to 5 L/min (**Fig. 6**). An oxygenator can be added if needed.[1,5,14]

TandemHeart support can provide more robust hemodynamic support than other tMCS options, including IABP. In a prospective study comparing outcomes and hemodynamic parameters for TandemHeart support with IABP among 42 patients, the cohort with TandemHeart support demonstrated a significantly higher increase in cardiac output and mean arterial pressure and a significant decrease in pulmonary capillary wedge pressure although overall 30-day survival and severe adverse events were no different among the groups.[19] In another study in which patients were randomized to either TandemHeart or IABP support, hemodynamic and metabolic parameters

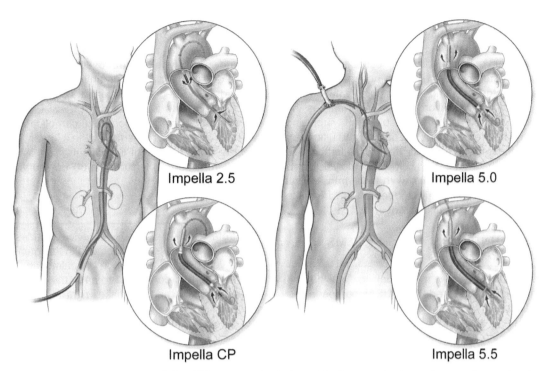

Fig. 5. Pictorial demonstration of the different Impella devices with the cannula situated across the aortic valve. (Reprinted with permission, Cleveland Clinic Foundation ©2023. All Rights Reserved.)

were improved more effectively with TandemHeart support, yet there was a higher rate of severe bleeding and limb ischemia among this cohort with a similar 30-day mortality rate.[20]

Placement of a TandemHeart system requires more expertise and time than some of the other support options owing to the need for a transseptal puncture. Positioning is key as migration

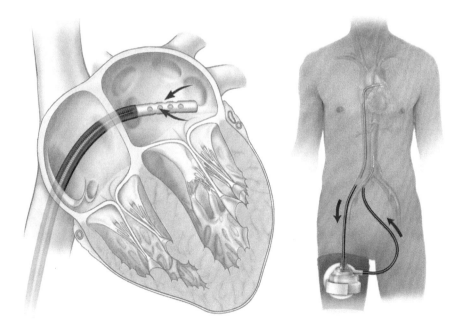

Fig. 6. TandemHeart illustration with trans-septal placement of cannula in left atrium. (Reprinted with permission, Cleveland Clinic Foundation ©2023. All Rights Reserved.)

of the cannula from the left atrium to the right atrium can result in immediate right-to-left shunting. In addition, flow support from the device depends on preload, afterload, cannula size, and appropriate positioning, which changes in any of these factors affecting the efficiency of the device. Right ventricle function is also important, as the right ventricle is responsible for supplying adequate preload to the left atrium, and ultimately the TandemHeart system. Other considerations to keep in mind are the risk of hemolysis, limb ischemia, complications with the trans-septal puncture, and air or thromboembolism from the device. Anticoagulation is required.[1,5,14]

RIGHT VENTRICLE SUPPORT SYSTEMS
Impella RP

As a catheter-based microaxial flow device, the Impella RP (Abiomed, MA, USA) pumps blood from the right atrium to the pulmonary artery, bypassing the right ventricle. The device decreases the right atrial pressure while increasing forward flow into the pulmonary artery and increasing preload to the left ventricle. It can provide up to 4 L/min of flow and, as of present, can only be placed via the femoral vein. Anticoagulation is required. Complications include limb ischemia, hemolysis, bleeding, and other vascular complications.[5,12]

The RECOVER RIGHT study assessed the safety and efficacy of the RP Impella as part of a prospective trial and demonstrated almost immediate hemodynamic improvement following device deployment, including an increase in cardiac index and decrease in central venous pressure. Survival rate at 30 days was 73.3% in this cohort, with the most common complications including bleeding and hemolysis. In a larger prospective cohort study of 60 patients, similar results were reported, including a 30-day survival rate of 72%.[21]

Protek Duo

The Protek Duo (LivaNova, UK) device includes a dual lumen, coaxial cannula located in the internal jugular vein with the distal tip in the pulmonary artery (**Fig. 7**). It is connected to an extracorporeal centrifugal pump and decreases right atrial pressure by directly venting the cavity while transferring blood to the pulmonary artery. This also allows for increased left ventricle preload. This device is able to augment cardiac output by 2 to 4 L/min, and unlike the Impella RP, an oxygenator can be connected to the Protek Duo circuit if needed.[5,10] Patients generally are able to ambulate with this device, and anticoagulation is required. Complications include bleeding, vascular injury, and hemolysis.[5]

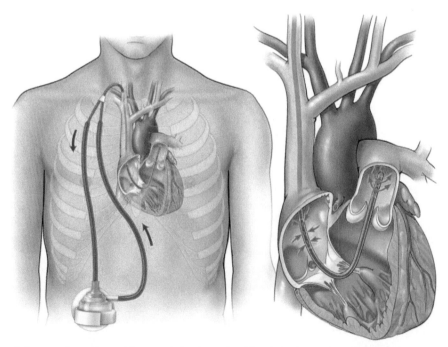

Fig. 7. Protek Duo configuration with cannula in the right side of the heart. (Reprinted with permission, Cleveland Clinic Foundation ©2023. All Rights Reserved.)

Data supporting its use are limited. The largest case series includes 17 patients from two centers with a mean length of support of 10.5 days. Although hemodynamic support was presumably achieved, only 23% of patients were successfully weaned from support, with the remainder necessitating longer-term surgical or durable right ventricular assist device support. Forty-one percent of patients in this cohort died, and complications were noted in 35% of the cohort, including injury to the internal jugular vein, intracranial bleeding, and bleeding at the catheter insertion site.[22]

BIVENTRICULAR SUPPORT SYSTEMS
CentriMag

The CentriMag(Abbott, Chicago, IL, USA) device is an extracorporeal centrifugal pump surgically implanted via median sternotomy and can supply isolated left, isolated right, or biventricular support based on its configuration (**Fig. 8**). It has a magnetically levitated impeller which is thought to result in improved hemocompatibility by significantly reducing friction within the pump apparatus and ultimately resulting in less blood trauma. Anticoagulation is required, yet these devices are thought to be more forgiving than others if anticoagulation is interrupted. Up to 10 L/min of support can be provided, and patients can generally be mobilized with this device configuration. It currently is approved for up to 30 days of use.[5,9]

Data supporting the use of CentriMag devices are limited and primarily include case series or case reports from single centers. In one such retrospective series of 63 patients, those that required the use of CentriMag support were refractory to medical management, and 85% of those patients were treated by IABP therapy at the time of CentriMag implantation. The majority had an INTERMACS 1 profile, and despite the severity of disease, outcomes demonstrated that 74% of patients survived to hospital discharge with a 1-year survival rate of 68%; however, thromboembolic events occurred in 10 patients, with 6 of those being strokes.[23]

Venoarterial Extracorporeal Membrane Oxygenation

Allowing for full hemodynamic support, venoarterial extracorporeal membrane oxygenation (VA ECMO) diverts blood from a systemic vein and delivers oxygenated blood back into the systemic arterial circulation. VA ECMO cannulation can take place peripherally and therefore can be advantageous as it can be placed at bedside in an acutely decompensating patient. VA ECMO technology has been in existence for over 6 decades and allows for full hemodynamic support with a flow of up to 6 L/min.[1,5,9,10,14,24] National trends demonstrate a substantial increase in its use, and VA ECMO is generally reserved for patients with refractory shock with biventricular dysfunction.[1,24] Important considerations to keep in mind with VA ECMO, similar to other tMCS options, is ensuring that an appropriate "exit strategy" exists considering VA ECMO provides full circulatory and respiratory support. There is no clear society-endorsed evidence-based guideline on the use of VA ECMO or in the selection of which patients are likely to benefit; therefore, multidisciplinary decision-making is crucial.[1,2,9] Different risk scores have been proposed to assess the likelihood to hospital discharge, including the PRESERVE, SAVE, and the simple cardiac ECMO scores.[25-27]

Cannulation sites typically include the femoral vein and femoral artery, yet utilization of the internal jugular vein and axillary artery can allow for

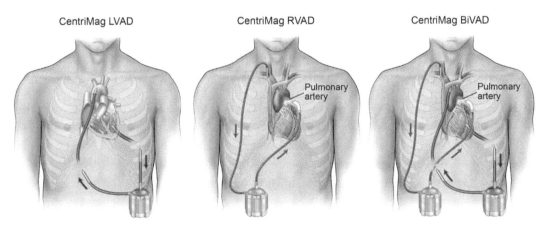

CentriMag LVAD   CentriMag RVAD   CentriMag BiVAD

Fig. 8. CentriMag illustration with various cannulation options allowing for LVAD, RVAD, or BiVAD support. (Reprinted with permission, Cleveland Clinic Foundation ©2023. All Rights Reserved.)

patient mobilization. An oxygenator can also be added to the circuit (**Fig. 9**). Furthermore, the use of an antegrade perfusion cannula is recommended to prevent limb ischemia. In addition, in the context of higher afterload, venting the left ventricle with either an Impella device or IABP may be important. The increase in arterial afterload can result in left ventricular distension and ultimately pulmonary edema, and a device to help decompress the left ventricle may be needed to prevent such events.[1,5,9,10,14,24] Serial evaluations of right radial artery blood gases is also important and considered standard for monitoring potential north-south syndrome.[24] Complications include bleeding, hemolysis, limb ischemia, and other vascular issues.[1,5,9,10,14,24]

Most data supporting the use of VA ECMO stem from registry or retrospective observational studies. No prospective randomized controlled trial exists in evaluating its efficacy, likely owing to the logistical and ethical issues involved with such studies among patients already refractory to other therapies.[24] The Extracorporeal Life Support Organization registry has evaluated over 15,000 patients since 1990 and demonstrated an approximate 40% survival rate to hospital discharge among patients on VA ECMO.[28] Other data have demonstrated a 6-month survival rate of only 30%. In another series, among patients in whom VA ECMO is used for cardiac arrest, the survival rate is 29%.[24] Noncardiac end-organ failure is associated with worse outcomes; therefore, this needs to be taken into account when selecting patients. Ideally, VA ECMO should be used before end-organ failure begins as this results in better outcomes.[2,9,10,24]

Device Transitions

An important ongoing multidisciplinary discussion piece that should start on day one of therapy and continue throughout its course is when to transition or wean device support.[11] Cardiogenic shock is a very dynamic process with various moving pieces, and it is imperative to ensure appropriate tailoring of therapy is achieved.[1,2,7,10] A ventricle-specific unloading strategy is recommended with continued evaluation of the underlying cardiogenic phenotype and what type of support, whether univentricular or biventricular, is needed. Wean attempts should be assessed daily, and a wean success is defined as clinical stability at low levels of device support, while meeting a set of hemodynamic, metabolic, and echocardiographic parameters.[11]

Just as importantly, it is important to discuss the decision on when to withhold support, or even escalation or support, or decide on when to withdraw support. Temporary mechanical circulatory support increases cardiac output yet generally does not address the underlying mechanism resulting in shock; therefore, ongoing discussions regarding support are needed. Numerous ethical and legal dilemmas surround the use of tMCS, and these types of discussions are important among all individuals involved in the patient's care. The emotional and ethical challenges facing health care providers, surrogate decision-makers, and families can impact decision-making. Oftentimes, the patient is unable to participate in such conversations, adding an additional layer of complexity. One of the most complex ethical and clinical paradigms is uncertainty, including uncertainty involving the patient's inherent

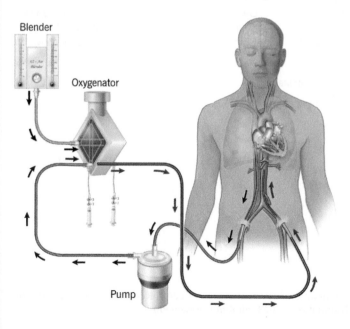

Fig. 9. Venoarterial extracorporeal membrane oxygenation illustration with peripheral cannulation. (Reprinted with permission, Cleveland Clinic Foundation ©2023. All Rights Reserved.)

Blender

Oxygenator

Pump

decision-making capacity, uncertainty involving the intended use of tMCS, and uncertainty involving the clinical outcome.[29,30] In one retrospective case series of almost 800 patients supported by Centri-Mag or VA ECMO support systems, tMCS was withdrawn in 22.4% of patients, and only 3.4% of patients possessed the capacity to participate in these discussions, underscoring the difficulty in end-of-life decision-making. Palliative care and ethics team involvement can be valuable in these circumstances.[30]

SUMMARY

As tMCS is used more widely, it becomes important to be able to identify patients that would benefit from such support. Cardiogenic shock results in high morbidity and mortality, and early recognition with early implementation of support is key. Defining the phenotype of cardiogenic shock, whether univentricular or biventricular support is needed, is a necessity in helping identify what type of support system best fits the needs of an individual patient, while also recognizing that hemodynamic phenotypes of cardiogenic shock can be fluid. The decision for device selection should be based on the individual patient's needs and comfort level of the clinical team. Most data supporting the use of tMCS have mixed results and generally stem from limited studies yet are also likely a result of very heterogeneous patient populations and life-threatening physiologic state seen among patients with cardiogenic shock.

Temporary mechanical circulatory support offers short-term hemodynamic support among a wide array of patients and can be utilized anywhere from hours to weeks, yet understanding the destination of this therapy is important. Decisions to initiate and escalate therapies require a comprehensive assessment in a multidisciplinary approach, including that of a formalized shock team. Temporary mechanical circulatory support offers lifesaving interventions to patients with cardiogenic shock refractory to medical therapy and will continue to play an important role as the technology continues to evolve.

CLINICS CARE POINTS

- Cardiogenic shock is a multi-organ system pathology that carries a high mortality rate as a result of tissue hypoperfusion.
- Prompt recogniition is key and defining a patient's hemodynamic profile helps to understand the phenotype of cardiogenic shock.

- Multi-disciplinary shock teams should be utilized and on-going evaluations for the need of temporary mechanical circulatory support should be discussed early on.
- A wide array of temporary mechanical circulatory support options are available and selection should be individualized.

DISCLOSURE

The authors have nothing to disclose.

REFERENCES

1. Combes A, Price S, Slutsky AS, et al. Temporary circulatory support for cardiogenic shock. Lancet 2020;396(10245):199–212.
2. Geller BJ, Sinha SS, Kapur NK, et al. Escalating and de-escalating temporary mechanical circulatory support in cardiogenic shock: a scientific statement from the American Heart Association. Circulation 2020;146(6):e50–68.
3. Ouweneel DM, Eriksen E, Sjauw KD, et al. Percutaneous mechanical circulatory support versus intra-aortic balloon pump in cardiogenic shock after acute myocardial infarction. J Am Coll Cardiol 2017;69:278–87.
4. Thiele H, Akin I, Sandri M, et al. PCI strategies in patients with acute myocardial infarction and cardiogenic shock. N Engl J Med 2017;377:2419–32.
5. Arora S, Atreya A, Birati E, et al. Temporary mechanical circulatory support as bridge to heart transplant or durable left ventricular assist device. Interv Cardiol Clin 2021;10(2):235–49.
6. Snipelisky D, Fudim M, Perez A, et al. Expected vs actual outcomes of elective initiation of inotropic therapy during heart failure hospitalization. Mayo Clin Proc Innov Qual Outcomes 2020;4(5):529–36.
7. Obradovic D, Freund A, Feistritzert HJ, et al. Temporary mechanical circulatory support in cardiogenic shock. Prog Cardiovasc Dis 2021;69:35–46.
8. Snipelisky, Chaudhry SP, Stewart GC. The many faces of heart failure. Card Electrophysiol Clin 2019;11(1):11–20.
9. Baran DA, Jaiswal A, Hennig F, et al. Temporary mechanical circulatory support: devices, outcomes, and future directions. J Heart Lung Transplant 2022;41(6):678–91.
10. Jiritano F, Coco VL, Matteucci M, et al. Temporary mechanical circulatory support in acute heart failure. Card Fail Rev 2020;16(6):e01.
11. Randhawa VK, Al-Fares A, Tong MZY, et al. A pragmatic approach to weaning temporary mechanical circulatory support: a state-of-the-art review. JACC Heart Fail 2021;9(9):664–73.

12. Salter BS, Gross CR, Weiner MM, et al. Temporary mechanical circulatory support devices: practical considerations for all stakeholders. Nat Rev Cardiol 2023;20:263–77.

13. Vieira JL, Ventrua HO, Mehra MR. Mechanical circulatory support devices in advanced heart failure: 2020 and beyond. Prog Cardiovasc Dis 2020; 63(5):630–9.

14. Marbach JA, Chewich H, Miyashita S, et al. Temporary mechanical circulatory support devices: updates from recent studies. Curr Opin Cardiol 2021; 36(4):375–83.

15. Bhimaraj A, Agrawal T, Duran A, et al. Percutaneous left axillary artery placement of intra-aortic balloon pump in advanced heart failure patients. JACC Heart Fail 2020;8(4):313–23.

16. Thiele H, Zeymer U, Neumann FJ, et al. Intraaortic balloon support for myocardial infarction with cardiogenic shock. N Engl J Med 2012;367(14):1287–96.

17. Hritani AW, Wani AS, Olet S, et al. Secular trend in the sure and implantation of Impella in high-risk percutaneous coronary intervention and cardiogenic shock: a real-word experience. J Invasive Cardiol 2019;31(9):e265–70.

18. Seese L, Hickey G, Keebler ME, et al. Direct bridging to cardiac transplantation with the surgically implanted Impella 5.0 device. Clin Transplant 2020;34(3):e13818.

19. Burkhoff D, Cohen H, Brunckhorst C, et al. A randomized multicenter clinical study to evaluate the safety and efficacy of the TandemHeart percutaneous ventricular assist device versus conventional therapy with intaaortic balloon pumping for treatment of cardiogenic shock. Am Heart J 2006; 152(3):469:e1–e8.

20. Thiele H, Sick P, Boudriot E, et al. Randomized comparison of intra-aortic balloon support with a percutaneous left ventricular assist device in patients with revascularized acute myocardial infarction complicated by cardiogenic shock. Eur Heart J 2005;26(13):1276–83.

21. Anderson MB, Goldstein J, Milano C, et al. Benefits of a novel percutaneous ventricular assist device for right heart failure: the prospective RECOVER RIGHT study of the Impella RP device. J Heart Lung Transplant 2015;34(12):1549–60.

22. Ravichandran AK, Baran DA, Stelling K, et al. Outcomes with the Tandem Protea Duo dual-lumen percutaneous right ventricular assist device. ASAIO J 2018;64(4):570–2.

23. Mehta V, Venkateswaran RV. Outcome of CentriMage extracorporeal mechanical circulatory support use in cardiogenic shock (INTERMACS 1) patients. Indian J Thorac Cardiovasc Surg 2020; 36(Supple 2):265–74.

24. Rao P, Khalpey Z, Smith R, et al. Venoarterial extracorporeal membrane oxygenation for cardiogenic shock and cardiac arrest. Circ Heart Failure 2018; 11(9):e004905.

25. Fisser C, Rincon-Gutierrez LA, Enger TB, et al. Validation of prognostic score in extracorporeal life support: a multi-centric retrospective study. Membranes 2021;11(2):84.

26. Schmidt M, Burell A, Roberts L, et al. Predicting survival of ECMO for refractory cardiogenic shock: the survival after veno-arterial ECMO (SAVE)-score. Eur Heart J 2015;36(33):2246–56.

27. Peigh G, Cavarocchi Nm, Keith SW, et al. Simple new risk score model for adult cardiac extracorporeal membrane oxygenation: simple cardiac ECMO score. J Surg Res 2015;198(2):273–9.

28. Paden ML, Conrad SA, Rycus PT, et al. Extracorporeal life support Organization registry report 2012. ASAIO J 2013;59(3):202–10.

29. Jaramillo C, Braus N. How should ECMO initiation and withdrawal decisions be shared? AMA J Ethics 2019;21(5):e387–93.

30. Carey MR, Tong W, Godfrey S, et al. Withdrawal of temporary mechanical circulatory support in patients with capacity. J Pain Symptom Manage 2022;63(3):387–94.

When all Else Fails, Try This

The HeartMate III Left Ventricle Assist Device

Abbas Bitar, MD*, Keith Aaronson, MD

KEYWORDS

- Left ventricle assist device • HeartMate III • Hemocompatibility-related adverse events
- Heart failure

KEY POINTS

- Continuous flow left ventricle assist devices (LVADs) improve survival and quality of life among patients with advanced heart failure.
- HeartMate III LVAD was designed to provide a better hemocompatibility profile than HeartMate II and HeatWare LVAD.
- Patients implanted with a HeartMate III have less hemocompatibility-related adverse events such as pump thrombosis and strokes.

INTRODUCTION

Heart failure (HF) is a global pandemic affecting more than 23 million adults worldwide.[1] It is estimated that more than 6 million American adults have HF.[1] HF is a progressive disease with an estimated 50% mortality within 5 years of diagnosis. The use of renin angiotensin blocking agents, sodium glucose cotransporter-2 inhibitors, resynchronization therapy, and defibrillator has improved overall survival. Nevertheless, it is estimated that 250,000 to 300,000 patients aged younger than 75 years suffer from advanced HF, defined as New York Heart Association (NYHA) class IIIB or IV, which is refractory to optimal medical therapy.[2] Patients with advanced HF have a 25% to 50% 1-year mortality.[1,3] Heart transplant remains the gold standard for patients with advanced HF. With increased hepatitis C donor utilization, donation after cardiac death and increased use of older donor heart, the number of heart transplant in the United Stated has increased during the past decade. Nevertheless, the number of patients with advanced HF surpasses current donor organ availability.[4] Left ventricle assist device (LVAD) were initially implanted in subjects with advanced HF presenting with cardiogenic shock as a bridge to transplantation or recovery. The advent of a more durable, smaller continuous flow pump (CF) with better hemocompatibility profile has led to the use of LVAD in a broader population during the past couple of decades. LVAD therapy improves survival and quality of life but continues to be associated with significant LVAD-related adverse events.[5] The aim of the current review is to provide an update on the indications, contraindications, and associated adverse events for LVAD support with a summary of the current outcomes data.

PATIENT SELECTION AND TIMING

More than 25,000 patients have undergone primary isolated CF-LVAD in the United States between 2010 and 2019 with now more than 3000 LVAD implant each year.[5] LVAD were initially used for a short period as bridge to heart transplant (BTT).[6] The REMATCH trial, published in 2001, demonstrated that LVAD use in patients with advanced HF not eligible for transplant

Department of Internal Medicine, Division of Cardiovascular Medicine, University of Michigan, Cardiovascular Center, 1500 East Medical Center Drive SPC 5853, Ann Arbor, MI 48109, USA
* Corresponding author.
E-mail address: abbitar@med.umich.edu

Cardiol Clin 41 (2023) 593–602
https://doi.org/10.1016/j.ccl.2023.06.009
0733-8651/23/© 2023 Elsevier Inc. All rights reserved.

reduced mortality (RR 0.52; 95% CI 0.34–0.78, P = .001) when compared with optimal medical therapy at 1 year of follow-up.[7] Since then, an increasing number of patients ineligible for transplant have received an LVAD as a permanent therapy referred as destination therapy (DT).[5] Patients receiving an LVAD who are initially ineligible for transplant due to a reversible comorbid condition that might improve with hemodynamic support, are designated as bridge to candidacy (BTC).[5]

During the last decade, there has been a change in the type of CF-LVAD type implanted. The HeartMate II LVAD (Abbott, Chigao, IL, USA) an axial flow pump was the first CF-LVAD approved by the Food and Drug Administration (FDA) as BTT in 2008 and DT in 2010. Subsequently, HeartWare, a centrifugal with hydromagnetic levitation (HVAD, Medtronic, Minnesota, MN, USA), was FDA approved as BTT and DT in 2012 and 2017, respectively. And most recently, HeartMate III (HMIII) (Abbott, Chicago, IL, USA), another centrifugal pump with improved hemocompatibility profile that is fully magnetically levitated, was FDA approved as BTT and DT in 2017 and 2018, respectively (**Fig. 1**). HMIII is currently the only commercially available LVAD in the United States after Medtronic stopped sales of HVAD in 2021 due to increased incidence of pump thrombosis and neurologic events.[8]

Between 2010 and 2019, 21.9%, 26.9%, and 50.5% of total CF-LVAD implanted were BTT, BTC, and DT, respectively. In 2019, more than 70% of LVAD implant were DT and less than 10% were BTT.[5] This shift in implant strategy can be attributed to the 2018 new heart allocation system, increased number of DT LVAD implantation center without heart transplant, and improved overall outcomes after LVAD implant.[5,9]

The ideal timing for LVAD implantation remains a challenge. Several prognostic risk scores such as the Seattle Heart Failure Model, Heart Failure Survival Score, Meta-Analysis Global Group in Chronic Heart Failure, incorporate various clinical and biochemical measurements to predict survival and risk of hospitalization in patients with chronic HF.[10–12] Moreover, mnemonics such as "I NEED HELP" is also used to initiate early referral for advanced therapies evaluation (**Table 1**).[13] The Interagency Registry for Mechanically Assisted Circulatory Support (INTERMACS) has developed 7 profiles that further stratify patients with advanced HF (NYHA IIIB and IV).[14] INTERMACS profile 1 to 3 describe inotrope dependent patients with INTERMACS 1 and 3 referring to patients with critical cardiogenic shock and stable on inotropic support respectively while profile 4 to 7 refer to non–inotrope-dependent patients with different level of HF symptoms limitations (**Table 2**).[14]

INDICATIONS AND CONTRAINDICATIONS FOR LEFT VENTRICLE ASSIST DEVICE THERAPY

LVAD and transplant evaluation share many indications. This includes severely reduced left

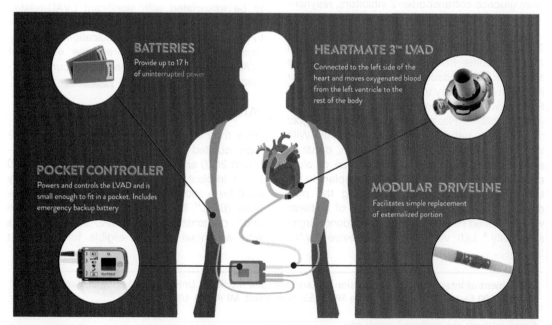

Fig. 1. HMIII left ventricular assist system components. (HeartMate and HeartMate 3 are trademarks of Abbott or its related companies. Reproduced with permission of Abbott, © 2023. All rights reserved.)

Table 1
Markers of advanced heart failure "I NEED HELP"

I	*I*notropes	Previous or ongoing requirement for dobutamine, milrinone, or dopamine
N	*N*YHA class/*N*atriuretic peptides	Persistent NYHA class III or IV and/or persistently elevated BNP or NT-proBNP
E	*E*nd-organ dysfunction	Worsening renal or liver dysfunction in the setting of HF
E	*E*jection fraction	Very-low LVEF of <20%
D	*D*efibrillator shocks	Recurrent appropriate defibrillator shocks
H	*H*ospitalizations	More than 1 heart hospitalization with HF in the last 12 mo
E	*E*dema/*E*scalating diuretics	Persistent fluid overload and/or increasing diuretic requirement
L	*L*ow blood pressure	Consistently low BP with systolic <90–100 mm Hg
P	*P*rognostic medication	Inability to up-titrate or need to stop/decrease ACEI, ARB, beta-blockers, ARNI or MRAs

Abbreviations: ACEI, angiotensin converting enzyme inhibitor; ARB, angiotensin receptor blocker; ARNI, angiotensin receptor-neprilysin inhibitor; BNP, brain natriuretic peptide; BP, blood pressure; MRA, mineralocorticoid receptor antagonist; NYHA, New York Heart Association.
From Baumwol J. "I Need Help"-A mnemonic to aid timely referral in advanced heart failure. J Heart Lung Transplant. 2017;36(5):593-594.

Table 2
The interagency registry for mechanically assisted circulatory support profiles

	Level	Hemodynamic Status	Time Frame for Intervention
1	Crash and burn	Persistent hypotension despite rapidly escalating support and eventually IABP and critical organ hypoperfusion	Within hours
2	Sliding on inotropes	Intravenous inotropic support with acceptable values of blood pressure and continuing deterioration in nutrition, renal function, or fluid retention	Within days
3	Dependent stability	Stability reached with mild-to-moderate doses of inotropes but demonstrated failure to wean from them due to hypotension, worsening symptoms, or progressive renal dysfunction	Elective over weeks or months
4	Frequent flyer	Possible weaning of inotropes but experiencing recurrent relapses, usually fluid retention	Elective over weeks or months
5	Housebound	Severely limited functional capacity: comfortable at rest with some volume overload and often with some renal dysfunction	Variable urgency, dependent on nutrition and organ function
6	Walking wounded	Less severely limited functional capacity and lack of volume overload	Variable urgency, dependent on nutrition and organ function
7	Placeholder	Patient without current or recent unstable fluid balance. NYHA class III	Not currently indicated

Abbreviations: IABP, intra-aortic balloon pump; NYHA, New York Heart Association.[14]
Adapted from Stevenson LW, Pagani FD, Young JB, et al. INTERMACS profiles of advanced heart failure: the current picture. J Heart Lung Transplant. 2009;28(6):535-541.

ventricle ejection fraction (LVEF <25%), intolerance of medical therapy, hypotension defined as a systolic blood pressure (SBP) of less than 90 mm Hg, worsening renal function, frequent and/or prolonged HF hospitalizations, and reduced maximal or submaximal exercise performance on a cardiopulmonary stress test defined as peak oxygen consumption (PVO_2) of less than 12 to 14 mL/kg/min with a respiratory exchange ratio of more than 1.05 or a minute ventilation/carbon dioxide (VE/VCO_2) slope of more than 35 with a submaximal stress test.[15–17] Cardiogenic shock defined as an SBP less than 90 mm Hg with a cardiac index (CI) of 1.8 L/min/m^2 off inotropes (CI < 2 L/min/m^2 on inotropes) in setting of elevated left-sided filling pressure (pulmonary capillary wedge pressure [PCWP] greater than 15 mm Hg) is another indication for advanced HF therapies evaluation. It is worth noting that certain absolute contraindications for heart transplant such as recent history of cancer, pulmonary hypertension with elevated and irreversible pulmonary vascular resistance and active tobacco use are not a contraindication for LVAD therapy.

Contraindication for LVAD therapy can be divided into medical and nonmedical. Medical contraindications can be cardiac or noncardiac.[17] Cardiac contraindication for LVAD therapy includes severe right ventricle dysfunction that will require permanent right ventricle assist device (RVAD) in a patient not eligible for transplant, refractory ventricular arrhythmias that cannot be controlled with antiarrhythmic or ablation and unfavorable cardiac anatomy (patients with hypertrophic/infiltrative cardiomyopathies, congenital heart disease with single ventricle), and patients with severe aortic insufficiency or earlier history of mechanical aortic valve replacement without a plan for bioprosthetic valve replacement or patch closure. Noncardiac medical contraindication includes history of active uncontrolled coagulopathy, inability to tolerate anticoagulation due to frequent episode of bleeding refractory to medical therapy, end-stage renal disease requiring hemodialysis, active malignancy with an expected survival of less than 2 years, severe obstructive or restrictive pulmonary disease, active uncontrolled infection, advanced age with frailty and severe cognitive impairment, or organic brain dysfunction affecting patient ability to manage their own care.[17] Nonadherence, untreated psychiatric illness, lack of caregiver support, and unaddressed alcohol and drug dependency are some of the major nonmedical contraindication for LVAD therapy that need to be addressed prepump implant by a multidisciplinary team consisting of a social worker, psychologist, and psychiatrist.[18]

OUTCOMES AFTER LEFT VENTRICLE ASSIST DEVICE IMPLANT

Despite increased preimplant illness severity, survival after CF-LVAD implantation has improved significantly between 2015 and 2019 when compared with prior era with a reported 1-year and 2-year survival of 82.3% and 73.1%, respectively.[5] Higher INTERMACS profile at time of implant is associated with improved survival. There is a stepwise drop in mortality moving from profile 1 to 2 to 3 (P < .0001) with overlapping survival curves for profile 3 and 4 to 7.[5] LVAD implant strategy correlate with overall survival. Bridge to transplant strategy is associated with higher 1-year survival compared with BTC and DT (86.8%, 83.8%, 80.1%, P < .0001). Postapproval registry for HMIII reported an 80% 2-year survival, which is comparable to 2 years postheart transplant outcome.[19] A recent 5-year analysis of the MOMENTUM 3 trial (In the Multicenter Study of MagLev Technology in Patients Undergoing Mechanical Circulatory Support Therapy with HeartMate III) reported an improved HMIII survival when compared with HMII (58.4% vs 43.7%, 95% CI 0.58–0.89, P = .003).[20] A similar HMIII 5-year survival (61%) was reported in a small European cohort.[21]

In addition to improved survival, CF-LVAD improves function capacity and quality of life. With CF-LVAD, 80% of patients had NYHA class I or II symptoms and sustained improvement in their 6-minute walking distance at 24 months of follow-up.[22–24] After LVAD implant patients benefited from an immediate and sustained improvement in their quality of life assessed using Minnesota Living with Heart Failure, Kansas City Cardiomyopathy, and EQ-5D questionnaires.[22–24]

ADVERSE EVENTS

Almost a third of patients after LVAD implant develop an early adverse event requiring hospitalization within 90 days after pump implant.[5] Some of the most common adverse events include hemocompatibility-related adverse event (HRAE), right ventricle failure, infection, aortic insufficiency (AI), and ventricular arrhythmias.

Hemocompatibility-related adverse events:

HRAEs include nonsurgical bleeding (NSB; gastrointestinal or other NSB episodes >30 days after implant), thromboembolic events such as suspected or confirmed pump thrombosis, arterial thromboembolism with or without organ involvement, and neurologic events such as ischemic or hemorrhagic strokes, transient ischemic attack, and seizures.[25] These events are associated with increased morbidity, mortality, worsening QOL, and increased health-care resource utilization.[5] The mechanisms for HRAEs are thought to be secondary to heightened systematic inflammation, microvascular dysfunction secondary to low pulsatile state, and increased shear stress from blood–pump interface leading to activation of different prothrombotic and proangiogenic pathways.[24] Moreover, current antithrombotic agents, warfarin (International normalized ratio [INR 2–3] and aspirin [81–325 mg/d]), that are used to mitigate thrombotic risk heighten bleeding risk.[25] For HMII and HVAD, the 1-year risk of pump thrombosis ranged from 8% to 10%, whereas only 1.4% of HMIII patients experienced pump thrombosis in the MOMENTUM 3 trial.[24]

Bleeding

Bleeding is one of the most common adverse events after LVAD implantation. Major bleeding accounts for 1.433 and 0.347 events per patient-years in the early (0–90 days) and later (>90 days) periods after CF-LVAD implant, respectively.[5] In the most recent INTERMACS report, gastrointestinal bleeding accounts for 50% of all bleeding events at 1 year of follow-up.[5] In the MOMENTUM 3 5-year follow-up trial, patients implanted with an HMIII (vs HMII) had lower NSB (0.430 vs 0.765 events/patient-years, $P < .001$) and gastrointestinal bleeding (GIB) events (0.252 vs 0.423 events/patient-years, $P < .001$).[20] The pathophysiology of NSB is complex and is thought to be secondary to overexpression of angiopoietin 2, part of a family of vascular growth factors that was found to be overexpressed and strongly associated with increased angiogenesis and increased risk of NSB.[26] Expression and release of Ang-2 is mediated through (1) increased degradation of high molecular weight von Willebrand Factor degradation preventing the formation of endothelial Weible Palade bodies; (2) tumor necrosis factor-α–mediated thrombin overexpression, pericyte apoptosis and downregulation of angiopoietin-1; (3) increased expression of hypoxia-induced factor 1a; and (4) activation of angiotensin type I receptor-mediated pathway.[26–29] Pathway-specific therapies such as angiotensin converting enzyme inhibitor (ACEI), angiotensin receptor blocker (ARB), digoxin, octreotide, and thalidomide have had some success in preventing and treating recurrent NSB secondary to angiodysplasia.[30–33] Antithrombotic reduction defined as lower INR goal and/or lower aspirin or aspirin-free antithrombotic regimen has been tested in few prospective and retrospective studies. Among HMIII recipients in the MOMENTUM 3 study, aspirin 81 mg daily was noninferior to 325 mg daily on a background of therapeutic anticoagulation (INR 2–3).[34] Aspirin-free antithrombotic regimen in HMIII LVAD recipients has been reported with favorable outcomes.[35,36] These observations created the foundation for the ARIES HMIII (Antiplatelet Removal and Hemocompatibility Events with the HeartMate III Pump) study, which randomized 628 HMIII receiving vitamin K antagonist to either a placebo or 100 mg of aspirin. The study completed enrollment in September 2022 and will be comparing survival free of HRAEs using a noninferiority analysis. Moreover, the MAGENTUM 1 (Minimal Anticoagulation Evaluation To Augment Hemocompatibility) study, a small pilot prospective study, demonstrated that less intense anticoagulation (INR goal of 1.5–2) was safe in 15 HMIII recipients and did not result in hemolysis, pump thrombosis, or a stroke at 6 months of follow-up.[37]

The role of direct oral anticoagulation agent is uncertain. In a small prospective open label single-center study, dabigatran was associated with increased thromboembolic events in HVAD recipients leading to early trial termination.[38] Currently, DOAC LVAD (Direct Oral Anti-Coagulant Apixaban in Left Ventricular Assist Devices) study is randomizing HMIII recipients to aspirin with either apixaban (5 mg bid) or warfarin (INR goal 2–2.5) and comparing survival free of HRAEs.

Strokes

Strokes, whether ischemic or hemorrhagic, are the most debilitating adverse events while on LVAD support. Ischemic strokes are thought to be embolic due to a clot formation in left atrial appendage, left ventricle, aortic valve, inside the pump housing, within the inflow, or outflow grafts. LVAD infection and uncontrolled hypertension have been identified as strong risk factors for both ischemic and hemorrhagic strokes.[39–41] Patients who experience frequent episodes of GIB after CF-LVAD have their antithrombic regimen intensity reduced, resulting in increased incidence of strokes.[41] Moreover, female gender, preimplant SBP, heparin-induced thrombocytopenia, intra-aortic balloon pump, and primary cardiac diagnosis are identified as risk factors for stroke after CF-LVAD implant.[41] In the most recent INTERMACS report, 87% and 76.3% of patients were stroke free at 1 and 3 years of follow-up, respectively.[5] On CF-LVAD support, survival at 6 months after an ischemic stroke is 66% and 35% after hemorrhagic stroke.[41] The proportion of patients dying of neurologic dysfunction has dropped over time, with about 15.6% of patients implanted between 2015 and 2019 dying because of a neurologic dysfunction compared with 19.1% of patients implanted between 2010 and 2014.[5] In the MOMENTUM 3 trial, the 2-year and 5-year stroke rates were twice as high in the HMII as the HMIII.[20,24] This reduction in neurologic events with HMIII can be attributed to improved pump hemocompatibility profile with less hemolysis, pump thrombosis, and increased health-care providers' knowledge in managing hypertension and CF-LVAD–related infection.

Aortic Insufficiency

An INTERMACS analysis reported that more than 50% of CF-LVAD have mild AI at 6 months of follow-up and 10% to 15% of patients without any AI before implant developed moderate-to-severe AI at 1-year of follow up.[42] Moreover, the rate of progression is higher among patients with preexisting AI.[42] LVAD will unload the left ventricle leading to reduced valve opening and closure. Increased hemodynamic stress on the aortic valve leaflet leads to frequent valvular endothelium microtrauma, adverse remodeling and degeneration, leaflet retraction and incompetent aortic valve leading to AI.[43] Risk factors associated with de novo or worsening AI include older age, female sex, hypertension, lower body mass index, moderate-to-severe mitral regurgitation, permanently closed aortic valve, preexisting AI, and DT strategy.[42,43] Moderate-to-severe AI results in inadequate left ventricle (LV) unloading leading to increased biventricular filling pressures, increased LV end diastolic dimension, worsening mitral regurgitation, reduced cardiac output, and organ perfusion.[43] Moderate-to-severe AI is associated with increased mortality and higher rehospitalization rate.[42] For patients with moderate-to-severe AI pre-LVAD, a bioprosthetic valve replacement, valve repair, or patching is recommended. For those who develop significant AI with refractory HF symptoms to volume status and pump speed optimization, AV replacement either surgically or through a transcatheter is recommended. Redo-sternotomy for AV replacement or repair is associated with increased mortality.[44] For high-risk surgical candidate transcatheter aortic valve replacement or percutaneous occlude devices have emerged as an effective alternative treatment option.[45,46]

Right Ventricle Failure

Approximately 20% to 40% of right ventricle (RV) systolic pressure and volume outflow results from LV contraction.[47] It is expected that all patients with severe LV dysfunction to have some degree of RV dysfunction. INTERMACS defines RV failure as persistent signs and symptoms of RV dysfunction evident by central venous pressure greater than 18 mm Hg with a CI less than 2 L/min/m^2 in the absence of an elevated PCWP (>18 mm Hg), cardiac tamponade, ventricular arrhythmias, or pneumothorax. RV failure after LVAD can be the result of an intrinsic RV dysfunction secondary to an underlying cardiomyopathy, patient comorbidities, and RV structural and functional changes after LVAD implant. LV unloading leads to a leftward shift in the interventricular septum leading to decreased septal contribution to RV contraction.[48] Moreover, increased RV preload can lead to RV enlargement, worsening RV mechanics, functional tricuspid regurgitation, increased wall stiffness, and decline in RV systolic function.[48] Perioperative insults such as vasoplegia, hypoxia, prolonged cardiopulmonary bypass, pulmonary hypertension, right coronary artery ischemia, and hypoxia have been identified as major contributor to RV failure after LVAD. Between 10% and 40% develop early RV failure within 2 weeks after LVAD implant.[49,50] In the MOMENTUM 3 trial, 34% of patients with HMIII developed RV failure and 4.1% required an RVAD.[24] Patients with lower INTERMACS profile are at increased risk for severe RV failure requiring RVAD support.[51] Additionally, RVAD insertion for acute RV failure is associated with increased mortality.[51] Nevertheless, early recognition of RV dysfunction with planned RVAD strategy may be associated with better outcome. Increased experience with percutaneous RVAD, such as Impella RP (Abiomed, Danvers, MA) and ProtkDuo (TandemLife, Pittsburgh, PA), for acute RV failure seems promising.[52] Chronic RV failure develops weeks to months after LVAD implant and is associated with worsening renal and hepatic function, diuretic resistance, frequent hospitalization, need for inotropes, and failure to thrive.

Several preoperative risk scores, echocardiographic, and hemodynamic parameters have been derived to predict risk of RV failure after LVAD implant. Most of those models were derived from single-center cohort with poor-to-modest discrimination value with different RV failure definitions.[53] Hemodynamic optimization during perioperative period with aggressive diuresis, inotropic support, use of inhaled or intravenous pulmonary vasodilators, maintenance of sinus rhythm, minimization of massive transfusion, prevention and minimization of respiratory and metabolic acidosis and adequate pump speed adjustment to maintain a midline interventricular septum position will help minimize acute RV failure after LVAD implant.

Furthermore, LVAD implant will reduce PCWP, RV afterload which overtime leads to improved RV function. Moreover, invasive hemodynamic optimization achieved through an invasive hemodynamic ramp test (pump speed is adjusted to achieve a CI > 2.2 L/min/m^2, PCWP <18 mm Hg, and RA <12 mm Hg) decreased both overall and HF hospitalization rates.[54]

Pump Infections

Ventricular assist device infection is defined by the International Society for Heart and Lung Transplantation (ISHLT) as "any infection that occurs in the presence of a ventricular assist device.[55] Infections after LVAD implant can be categorized as device specific (pump or cannula, pocket or driveline infection), device related (mediastinitis, infective endocarditis or blood stream infections), and non–device-related (pneumonia, cellulitis, urinary tract infection, and so forth).[56] LVAD infections are associated with significant mortality and morbidity. Older age, renal failure, prolonged LVAD support, diabetes mellitus, and malnutrition have been reported as risk factors for infections after LVAD implant.[55,57] Major infections account for most adverse events in the early and late phase, 1.349 and 0.440 events per patient-year, respectively, after CF-LVAD implant.[5] A similar trend was reported by the MOMENUM 3 5-year follow-up trial with both HMIII and HMII showing an elevated rate of major infection 0.515 and 0.551 event per patient-year (P = .25), respectively.[20] In the most recent INTERMACS analysis, only 59% and 46.4% of patients were free from infection at 1 and 2 years of follow-up.[5] Non–device-related infections account for most of the infection in the first 3 months after implant and driveline infections account for most of the infections thereafter.[5,58] Gram-positive cocci such as Staphylococcus aureus and Staphylococcus epidermis are the most common pathogens associated with driveline infections. Gram-negative rods such as Pseudomonas and Klebsiella, in addition to fungal infection, are less common organisms.[59] Meticulous driveline care by healthcare staff, patients, and caregivers by consistently securing drive line, preventing driveline pulling or twisting, and periodic driveline exit site cleaning are key to prevent any driveline-related infection.

Driveline and blood culture in addition to driveline ultrasound, computed tomography, and 18F-fluorodeoxyglucose positron emission tomography CT are used to identify the causative pathogen and extend of LVAD infection.[60] Treatment of LVAD infections depends on the causative microorganism and extent of infection. For patients with superficial driveline infection, usually a 10 to 14-day course of oral antibiotics is sufficient. For those with pocket infection, deep soft tissue infection or bacteremia, 6 to 8 weeks of intravenous antibiotics followed by suppressive antibiotic therapy is indicated. Patients with an abscess benefit from drainage and those with refractory driveline infection (in the absence of mediastinal involvement) benefit from either a partial or complete driveline relocation with omental wrapping.[61] Pump exchange is reserved for patients with persistent bacteremia and recurrent infection resistant to appropriate antibiotic therapy. Recurrent LVAD infection after pump exchange remains substantial. For those eligible for transplant, a higher listing status can prevent another sternotomy, decrease waitlist time, and provide a definitive treatment option for infection.

SUMMARY

With a limited donor pool for heart transplant, CF-LVAD therapy remains a lifesaving treatment option for patients with advanced HF. The development of smaller and more durable pumps with an improved hemocompatibility profile resulted in improved overall survival after CF-LVAD. Patients implanted with HMIII experienced less pump thrombosis and strokes in the MOMENTUM 3 trial at 2 and 5 years of follow-up. A fully implantable LVAD will contribute to a wider adoption among patients with advanced HF and will likely contribute to an even lower rate of infections after implant.

CLINICS CARE POINTS

- Heart failure is a progressive disease.
- For patients with advanced heart failure, LVAD therapy improves quality of life and survival.

DISCLOSURE

The author and his coauthor have nothing to disclose as it relate to this article.

REFERENCES

1. Tsao CW, Aday AW, Almarzooq ZI, et al. Heart disease and stroke statistics-2022 update: a report from the American heart association. Circulation 2022;145(8):e153–639.

2. Miller LW. Left ventricular assist devices are underutilized. Circulation 2011;123(14):1552–8 [discussion: 1558].

3. Gustafsson F, Rogers JG. Left ventricular assist device therapy in advanced heart failure: patient selection and outcomes. Eur J Heart Fail 2017;19(5): 595–602.

4. DeFilippis EM, Khush KK, Farr MA, et al. Evolving characteristics of heart transplantation donors and recipients: JACC focus seminar. J Am Coll Cardiol 2022;79(11):1108–23.

5. Molina EJ, Shah P, Kiernan MS, et al. The society of thoracic surgeons intermacs 2020 annual report. Ann Thorac Surg 2021;111(3):778–92.

6. Miller LW, Pagani FD, Russell SD, et al. Use of a continuous-flow device in patients awaiting heart transplantation. N Engl J Med 2007;357(9):885–96.

7. Rose EA, Gelijns AC, Moskowitz AJ, et al. Long-term use of a left ventricular assist device for end-stage heart failure. N Engl J Med 2001; 345(20):1435–43.

8. Potapov EV, Nersesian G, Lewin D, et al. Propensity score-based analysis of long-term follow-up in patients supported with durable centrifugal left ventricular assist devices: the EUROMACS analysis. Eur J Cardio Thorac Surg 2021;60(3): 579–87.

9. Brinkley DM, DeNofrio D, Ruthazer R, et al. Outcomes after continuous-flow left ventricular assist device implantation as destination therapy at transplant versus nontransplant centers. Circ Heart Fail 2018;11(3):e004384.

10. Levy WC, Mozaffarian D, Linker DT, et al. The Seattle Heart Failure Model: prediction of survival in heart failure. Circulation 2006;113(11):1424–33.

11. Aaronson KD, Schwartz JS, Chen TM, et al. Development and prospective validation of a clinical index to predict survival in ambulatory patients referred for cardiac transplant evaluation. Circulation 1997; 95(12):2660–7.

12. Pocock SJ, Ariti CA, McMurray JJ, et al. Predicting survival in heart failure: a risk score based on 39 372 patients from 30 studies. Eur Heart J 2013; 34(19):1404–13.

13. Baumwol J. "I Need Help"-A mnemonic to aid timely referral in advanced heart failure. J Heart Lung Transplant 2017;36(5):593–4.

14. Stevenson LW, Pagani FD, Young JB, et al. INTERMACS profiles of advanced heart failure: the current picture. J Heart Lung Transplant 2009;28(6): 535–41.

15. Heidenreich PA, Bozkurt B, Aguilar D, et al. AHA/ACC/HFSA guideline for the management of heart failure: a report of the American college of cardiology/American heart association joint committee on clinical practice guidelines. Circulation 2022; 145(18):e895–1032.

16. Mehra MR, Canter CE, Hannan MM, et al. The 2016 International Society for Heart Lung Transplantation listing criteria for heart transplantation: a 10-year update. J Heart Lung Transplant 2016;35(1): 1–23.

17. Cook JL, Colvin M, Francis GS, et al. Recommendations for the use of mechanical circulatory support: ambulatory and community patient care: a scientific statement from the American heart association. Circulation 2017;135(25):e1145–58.

18. Dew MA, DiMartini AF, Dobbels F, et al. The 2018 ISHLT/APM/AST/ICCAC/STSW recommendations for the psychosocial evaluation of adult cardiothoracic transplant candidates and candidates for long-term mechanical circulatory support. Psychosomatics 2018;59(5):415–40.

19. Mehra MR, Cleveland JC Jr, Uriel N, et al. Primary results of long-term outcomes in the MOMENTUM 3 pivotal trial and continued access protocol study phase: a study of 2200 HeartMate 3 left ventricular assist device implants. Eur J Heart Fail 2021;23(8): 1392–400.

20. Mehra MR, Goldstein DJ, Cleveland JC, et al. Five-year outcomes in patients with fully magnetically levitated vs axial-flow left ventricular assist devices in the MOMENTUM 3 randomized trial. JAMA 2022;328(12):1233–42.

21. Netuka I, Pya Y, Zimpfer D, et al. First 5-year multicentric clinical trial experience with the HeartMate 3 left ventricular assist system. J Heart Lung Transplant 2021;40(4):247–50.

22. Slaughter MS, Rogers JG, Milano CA, et al. Advanced heart failure treated with continuous-flow left ventricular assist device. N Engl J Med 2009; 361(23):2241–51.

23. Mehra MR, Goldstein DJ, Uriel N, et al. Two-year outcomes with a magnetically levitated cardiac pump in heart failure. N Engl J Med 2018;378(15):1386–95.

24. Mehra MR, Uriel N, Naka Y, et al. A fully magnetically levitated left ventricular assist device - final report. N Engl J Med 2019;380(17):1618–27.

25. Mehra MR. The burden of haemocompatibility with left ventricular assist systems: a complex weave. Eur Heart J 2019;40(8):673–7.

26. Tabit CE, Chen P, Kim GH, et al. Elevated angiopoietin-2 level in patients with continuous-flow left ventricular assist devices leads to altered angiogenesis and is associated with higher nonsurgical bleeding. Circulation 2016;134(2):141–52.

27. Kang J, Hennessy-Strahs S, Kwiatkowski P, et al. Continuous-flow LVAD support causes a distinct form of intestinal angiodysplasia. Circ Res 2017; 121(8):963–9.

28. Tabit CE, Coplan MJ, Chen P, et al. Tumor necrosis factor-alpha levels and non-surgical bleeding in continuous-flow left ventricular assist devices. J Heart Lung Transplant 2018;37(1):107–15.

29. Pichiule P, Chavez JC, LaManna JC. Hypoxic regulation of angiopoietin-2 expression in endothelial cells. J Biol Chem 2004;279(13):12171–80.

30. Shah KB, Gunda S, Emani S, et al. Multicenter evaluation of octreotide as secondary prophylaxis in patients with left ventricular assist devices and gastrointestinal bleeding. Circ Heart Fail 2017; 10(11).

31. Converse MP, Sobhanian M, Taber DJ, et al. Effect of angiotensin II inhibitors on gastrointestinal bleeding in patients with left ventricular assist devices. J Am Coll Cardiol 2019;73(14):1769–78.

32. Houston BA, Schneider AL, Vaishnav J, et al. Angiotensin II antagonism is associated with reduced risk for gastrointestinal bleeding caused by arteriovenous malformations in patients with left ventricular assist devices. J Heart Lung Transplant 2017; 36(4):380–5.

33. Vukelic S, Vlismas PP, Patel SR, et al. Digoxin is associated with a decreased incidence of angiodysplasia-related gastrointestinal bleeding in patients with continuous-flow left ventricular assist devices. Circ Heart Fail 2018;11(8):e004899.

34. Saeed O, Colombo PC, Mehra MR, et al. Effect of aspirin dose on hemocompatibility-related outcomes with a magnetically levitated left ventricular assist device: an analysis from the MOMENTUM 3 study. J Heart Lung Transplant 2020;39(6):518–25.

35. Consolo F, Raimondi Lucchetti M, Tramontin C, et al. Do we need aspirin in HeartMate 3 patients? Eur J Heart Fail 2019;21(6):815–7.

36. Lim HS, Ranasinghe A, Chue C, et al. Two-year outcome of warfarin monotherapy in HeartMate 3 left ventricular assist device: a single-center experience. J Heart Lung Transplant 2020;39(10): 1149–51.

37. Netuka I, Ivak P, Tucanova Z, et al. Evaluation of low-intensity anti-coagulation with a fully magnetically levitated centrifugal-flow circulatory pump-the MAGENTUM 1 study. J Heart Lung Transplant 2018; 37(5):579–86.

38. Andreas M, Moayedifar R, Wieselthaler G, et al. Increased thromboembolic events with dabigatran compared with vitamin K antagonism in left ventricular assist device patients: a randomized controlled pilot trial. Circ Heart Fail 2017;10(5):e003709.

39. Shah P, Birk SE, Cooper LB, et al. Stroke and death risk in ventricular assist device patients varies by ISHLT infection category: an INTERMACS analysis. J Heart Lung Transplant 2019;38(7):721–30.

40. Teuteberg JJ, Slaughter MS, Rogers JG, et al. The HVAD left ventricular assist device: risk factors for neurological events and risk mitigation strategies. JACC Heart Fail 2015;3(10):818–28.

41. Acharya D, Loyaga-Rendon R, Morgan CJ, et al. INTERMACS analysis of stroke during support with continuous-flow left ventricular assist devices: risk factors and outcomes. JACC Heart Fail 2017;5(10): 703–11.

42. Truby LK, Garan AR, Givens RC, et al. Aortic insufficiency during contemporary left ventricular assist device support: analysis of the INTERMACS registry. JACC Heart Fail 2018;6(11):951–60.

43. Bouabdallaoui N, El-Hamamsy I, Pham M, et al. Aortic regurgitation in patients with a left ventricular assist device: a contemporary review. J Heart Lung Transplant 2018;37(11):1289–97.

44. Atkins BZ, Hashmi ZA, Ganapathi AM, et al. Surgical correction of aortic valve insufficiency after left ventricular assist device implantation. J Thorac Cardiovasc Surg 2013;146(5):1247–52.

45. Yehya A, Rajagopal V, Meduri C, et al. Short-term results with transcatheter aortic valve replacement for treatment of left ventricular assist device patients with symptomatic aortic insufficiency. J Heart Lung Transplant 2019;38(9):920–6.

46. Phan K, Haswell JM, Xu J, et al. Percutaneous transcatheter interventions for aortic insufficiency in continuous-flow left ventricular assist device patients: a systematic review and meta-analysis. ASAIO J 2017;63(2):117–22.

47. Santamore WP, Dell'Italia LJ. Ventricular interdependence: significant left ventricular contributions to right ventricular systolic function. Prog Cardiovasc Dis 1998;40(4):289–308.

48. Houston BA, Shah KB, Mehra MR, et al. A new "twist" on right heart failure with left ventricular assist systems. J Heart Lung Transplant 2017;36(7):701–7.

49. Bellavia D, Iacovoni A, Scardulla C, et al. Prediction of right ventricular failure after ventricular assist device implant: systematic review and meta-analysis of observational studies. Eur J Heart Fail 2017;19(7): 926–46.

50. Logstrup BB, Nemec P, Schoenrath F, et al. Heart failure etiology and risk of right heart failure in adult left ventricular assist device support: the European Registry for Patients with Mechanical Circulatory Support (EUROMACS). Scand Cardiovasc J 2020; 54(5):306–14.

51. Kirklin JK, Pagani FD, Kormos RL, et al. Eighth annual INTERMACS report: special focus on framing the impact of adverse events. J Heart Lung Transplant 2017;36(10):1080–6.

52. Coromilas EJ, Takeda K, Ando M, et al. Comparison of percutaneous and surgical right ventricular assist device support after durable left ventricular assist device insertion. J Card Fail 2019;25(2):105–13.

53. Frankfurter C, Molinero M, Vishram-Nielsen JKK, et al. Predicting the risk of right ventricular failure in patients undergoing left ventricular assist device implantation: a systematic review. Circ Heart Fail 2020;13(10):e006994.

54. Imamura T, Jeevanandam V, Kim G, et al. Optimal hemodynamics during left ventricular assist device

support are associated with reduced readmission rates. Circ Heart Fail 2019;12(2):e005094.

55. Hannan MM, Husain S, Mattner F, et al. Working formulation for the standardization of definitions of infections in patients using ventricular assist devices. J Heart Lung Transplant 2011;30(4):375–84.

56. Holman WL, Kirklin JK, Naftel DC, et al. Infection after implantation of pulsatile mechanical circulatory support devices. J Thorac Cardiovasc Surg 2010; 139(6):1632–1636 e2.

57. Pienta MJ, Shore S, Watt TMF, et al. Patient factors associated with left ventricular assist device infections: a scoping review. J Heart Lung Transplant 2022;41(4):425–33.

58. Givertz MM, DeFilippis EM, Colvin M, et al. HFSA/SAEM/ISHLT clinical expert consensus document on the emergency management of patients with ventricular assist devices. J Heart Lung Transplant 2019;38(7):677–98.

59. Blanco-Guzman MO, Wang X, Vader JM, et al. Epidemiology of left ventricular assist device infections: findings from a large nonregistry cohort. Clin Infect Dis 2021;72(2):190–7.

60. Almarzooq ZI, Varshney AS, Vaduganathan M, et al. Expanding the scope of multimodality imaging in durable mechanical circulatory support. JACC Cardiovasc Imaging 2020;13(4):1069–81.

61. Pieri M, Scandroglio AM, Muller M, et al. Surgical management of driveline infections in patients with left ventricular assist devices. J Card Surg 2016;31(12):765–71.

UNITED STATES POSTAL SERVICE®
Statement of Ownership, Management, and Circulation
(All Periodicals Publications Except Requester Publications)

1. Publication Title	2. Publication Number	3. Filing Date
CARDIOLOGY CLINICS	000 – 701	9/18/2023

4. Issue Frequency	5. Number of Issues Published Annually	6. Annual Subscription Price
FEB, MAY, AUG, NOV	4	$377.00

7. Complete Mailing Address of Known Office of Publication (Not printer) (Street, city, county, state, and ZIP+4®)

ELSEVIER INC.
230 Park Avenue, Suite 800
New York, NY 10169

Contact Person
Malathi Samayan

Telephone (Include area code)
91-44-4299-4507

8. Complete Mailing Address of Headquarters or General Business Office of Publisher (Not printer)

ELSEVIER INC.
230 Park Avenue, Suite 800
New York, NY 10169

9. Full Names and Complete Mailing Addresses of Publisher, Editor, and Managing Editor (Do not leave blank)

Publisher (Name and complete mailing address)

Dolores Meloni, ELSEVIER INC.
1600 JOHN F KENNEDY BLVD. SUITE 1600
PHILADELPHIA, PA 19103-2899

Editor (Name and complete mailing address)

JOANNA COLLETT, ELSEVIER INC.
1600 JOHN F KENNEDY BLVD. SUITE 1600
PHILADELPHIA, PA 19103-2899

Managing Editor (Name and complete mailing address)

PATRICK MANLEY, ELSEVIER INC.
1600 JOHN F KENNEDY BLVD. SUITE 1600
PHILADELPHIA, PA 19103-2899

10. Owner (Do not leave blank. If the publication is owned by a corporation, give the name and address of the corporation immediately followed by the names and addresses of all stockholders owning or holding 1 percent or more of the total amount of stock. If not owned by a corporation, give the names and addresses of the individual owners. If owned by a partnership or other unincorporated firm, give its name and address as well as those of each individual owner. If the publication is published by a nonprofit organization, give its name and address.)

Full Name	Complete Mailing Address
WHOLLY OWNED SUBSIDIARY OF REED/ELSEVIER, US HOLDINGS	1600 JOHN F KENNEDY BLVD. SUITE 1600 PHILADELPHIA, PA 19103-2899

11. Known Bondholders, Mortgagees, and Other Security Holders Owning or Holding 1 Percent or More of Total Amount of Bonds, Mortgages, or Other Securities. If none, check box. ► ☐ None

Full Name	Complete Mailing Address
N/A	

12. Tax Status (For completion by nonprofit organizations authorized to mail at nonprofit rates) (Check one)
The purpose, function, and nonprofit status of this organization and the exempt status for federal income tax purposes:
☒ Has Not Changed During Preceding 12 Months
☐ Has Changed During Preceding 12 Months (Publisher must submit explanation of change with this statement)

PS Form 3526, July 2014 [Page 1 of 4 (see instructions page 4)] PSN: 7530-01-000-9931 PRIVACY NOTICE: See our privacy policy on www.usps.com.

---

13. Publication Title	14. Issue Date for Circulation Data Below
CARDIOLOGY CLINICS	AUGUST 2023

15. Extent and Nature of Circulation		Average No. Copies Each Issue During Preceding 12 Months	No. Copies of Single Issue Published Nearest to Filing Date
a. Total Number of Copies (Net press run)		144	136
b. Paid Circulation (By Mail and Outside the Mail)	(1) Mailed Outside-County Paid Subscriptions Stated on PS Form 3541 (Include paid distribution above nominal rate, advertiser's proof copies, and exchange copies)	78	75
	(2) Mailed In-County Paid Subscriptions Stated on PS Form 3541 (Include paid distribution above nominal rate, advertiser's proof copies, and exchange copies)	0	0
	(3) Paid Distribution Outside the Mails Including Sales Through Dealers and Carriers, Street Vendors, Counter Sales, and Other Paid Distribution Outside USPS®	47	40
	(4) Paid Distribution by Other Classes of Mail Through the USPS (e.g., First-Class Mail®)	10	12
c. Total Paid Distribution (Sum of 15b (1), (2), (3), and (4))	►	135	127
d. Free or Nominal Rate Distribution (By Mail and Outside the Mail)	(1) Free or Nominal Rate Outside-County Copies Included on PS Form 3541	8	8
	(2) Free or Nominal Rate In-County Copies Included on PS Form 3541	0	0
	(3) Free or Nominal Rate Copies Mailed at Other Classes Through the USPS (e.g., First-Class Mail)	0	0
	(4) Free or Nominal Rate Distribution Outside the Mail (Carriers or other means)	1	1
e. Total Free or Nominal Rate Distribution (Sum of 15d (1), (2), (3) and (4))	►	9	9
f. Total Distribution (Sum of 15c and 15e)	►	144	136
g. Copies not Distributed (See Instructions to Publishers #4 (page #3))	►	0	0
h. Total (Sum of 15f and g)	►	144	136
i. Percent Paid (15c divided by 15f times 100)	►	93.75%	93.38%

* If you are claiming electronic copies, go to line 16 on page 3. If you are not claiming electronic copies, skip to line 17 on page 3.

PS Form 3526, July 2014 (Page 2 of 4)

16. Electronic Copy Circulation	Average No. Copies Each Issue During Preceding 12 Months	No. Copies of Single Issue Published Nearest to Filing Date
a. Paid Electronic Copies ►		
b. Total Paid Print Copies (Line 15c) + Paid Electronic Copies (Line 16a) ►		
c. Total Print Distribution (Line 15f) + Paid Electronic Copies (Line 16a) ►		
d. Percent Paid (Both Print & Electronic Copies) (16b divided by 16c × 100) ►		

☒ I certify that 50% of all my distributed copies (electronic and print) are paid above a nominal price.

17. Publication of Statement of Ownership

☒ If the publication is a general publication, publication of this statement is required. Will be printed
in the __NOVEMBER 2023__ issue of this publication.

☐ Publication not required.

18. Signature and Title of Editor, Publisher, Business Manager, or Owner

Malathi Samayan

Malathi Samayan - Distribution Controller

Date
9/18/2023

I certify that all information furnished on this form is true and complete. I understand that anyone who furnishes false or misleading information on this form or who omits material or information requested on the form may be subject to criminal sanctions (including fines and imprisonment) and/or civil sanctions (including civil penalties).

PS Form 3526, July 2014 (Page 3 of 4) PRIVACY NOTICE: See our privacy policy on www.usps.com

Moving?

Make sure your subscription moves with you!

To notify us of your new address, find your **Clinics Account Number** (located on your mailing label above your name), and contact customer service at:

Email: journalscustomerservice-usa@elsevier.com

800-654-2452 (subscribers in the U.S. & Canada)
314-447-8871 (subscribers outside of the U.S. & Canada)

Fax number: 314-447-8029

Elsevier Health Sciences Division
Subscription Customer Service
3251 Riverport Lane
Maryland Heights, MO 63043

*To ensure uninterrupted delivery of your subscription, please notify us at least 4 weeks in advance of move.

Printed and bound by CPI Group (UK) Ltd, Croydon, CR0 4YY

03/10/2024

01040365-0009